Contemporary Diagnosis and Management of

Antimicrobial-Resistant Bacteria®

Gary A. Noskin, MD

Associate Professor of Medicine

Division of Infectious Diseases

*Northwestern University's
  Feinberg School of Medicine*

*Medical Director, Healthcare Epidemiology
  and Quality*

Northwestern Memorial Hospital

Chicago, Illinois

First Edition
Published by Handbooks in Health Care Co.,
Newtown, Pennsylvania, USA

International Standard Book Number: 1-931981-50-7

Library of Congress Catalog Card Number: 2005938799

Web site: www.HHCbooks.com

Table of Contents

This book has been prepared and is presented as a service to the medical community. The information provided reflects the knowledge, experience, and personal opinions of the author, Gary A. Noskin, MD, Associate Professor of Medicine, Division of Infectious Diseases, Northwestern University's Feinberg School of Medicine, and Medical Director, Healthcare Epidemiology and Quality, Northwestern Memorial Hospital, Chicago, Illinois.

This book is not intended to replace or to be used as a substitute for the complete prescribing information prepared by each manufacturer for each drug. Because of possible variations in drug indications, in dosage information, in newly described toxicities, in drug/drug interactions, and in other items of importance, reference to such complete prescribing information is definitely recommended before any of the drugs discussed are used or prescribed.

Acknowledgment

Dee A. Simmons, a medical writer, contributed to the research and writing of this book.

 **Chapter 1**

Introduction:
The Problem of Resistance

O nce heralded as a 'miracle drug,' penicillin was the first antibiotic in the war against infectious disease. Its power to cure skin and soft tissue infections, bacteremias, and pneumonias made it a vital ally during World War II, and spurred public interest in the drug. As penicillin gained a reputation as a cure-all, pharmaceutical companies responded to public demand and produced throat sprays, cough lozenges, mouthwashes, soaps, and other products containing penicillin, as well as oral and injectable forms of the drug. From its introduction in 1942 to the mid-1950s, penicillin was available without a prescription as an over-the-counter medication.[1]

Alexander Fleming, the bacteriologist who discovered penicillin, recognized the potential for misuse and warned that misuse could result in the development of mutant forms of bacteria that were resistant to the drug. In an interview in the *New York Times* in 1945, Fleming cautioned, "The greatest possibility of evil in self-medication is the use of too-small doses so that instead of clearing up infection, the microbes are educated to resist penicillin and a host of penicillin-fast organisms is bred out which can be passed to other individuals and from them to others until they reach someone who gets a septicemia or a pneumonia, which penicillin cannot save."[2]

Fleming's words proved true, not just for penicillin but for each new antibiotic subsequently developed. One by

one, antibiotics have been defeated or rendered less effective by resistant strains of bacteria, and a crisis looms
in the near future.

History of Antibiotics

Bacteria are the oldest known living things on earth,
dating back at least 3.5 billion years.[1] They are found on
every surface of our environment and on and in our bodies. But until the microscope was discovered in 1674 by
a Dutch dry goods merchant, Anton van Leeuwenhoek,
these single-celled microbes and their power to cause
disease remained hidden.[2] It took another 200 years to
make the connection between these tiny organisms and
the diseases they cause. It was a Frenchman, Louis Pas-
teur, who proposed the 'germ theory' of disease, suggest-
ing that bacteria were disease agents. Once the germ
theory of infection gained favor in the medical community, the search was under way for agents that would kill
these microscopic organisms.

In 1881, Robert Koch developed a gelatin and agar
medium on which bacteria could multiply.[2] Different
bacterial types could be identified, and substances that
might inhibit their growth could be tested on the plate.

A Danish physician, Hans Christian Gram, further contributed to the developing science of microbiology. He noticed that when bacteria were treated with a solution that
stained them a blue-purple color, some lost the dye when
washed with acetone, while others remained blue-purple.
Those that retained the dark purple color he called 'stain
positive;' those that lost the color and were subsequently
treated with a lighter dye, which turned them pink, were
called 'stain negative.'[1,2] Eventually, these terms became
gram-positive and *gram-negative*. Gram staining conve-
niently divided bacteria into two classes, each with distinctive traits. Among the gram-positives are *Staphylococcus,*
Streptococcus, Enterococcus, Bacillus, Listeria,
Clostridium, and *Mycoplasma.* The gram-positives have

single-layer cell walls, with the exception of the *Myco-plasma*, which has no cell walls. The gram-negatives, including *Escherichia coli, Acinetobacter baumannii, Pseudomonas aeruginosa, Salmonella, Moraxella, Helicobacter, Klebsiella pneumoniae,* and many others, have two-layer cell membranes but no cell walls.[3] The specific traits associated with each gram-stained class proved to be valuable in developing antibiotics to penetrate the bacteria's defenses.

Evidence unearthed in archaeologic digs and from ancient writings points to the early use of molds, other naturally occurring substances, and even soil, for healing wounds. In his studies, Koch noticed that pathogenic bacteria died when covered with soil. Researchers began to study soil, searching for entities that would inhibit or kill bacteria.

In 1888, an in vitro experiment in Germany revealed that a blue pigment from the bacterium *Bacillus pyocyaneus* (today called *P aeruginosa*) inhibited growth of other bacteria in the test tube.[2] Further clinical studies indicated that the substance, which was termed 'pyocyanase,' also killed the pathogens that caused anthrax, diphtheria, typhoid fever, plague, and skin abscesses, as well as inhibited bacterial growth. Out of the laboratory, however, pyocyanase proved toxic to patients and could only be used topically.

In 1910, in his search for a cure for African sleeping sickness, Paul Ehrlich developed a drug, salvarsan, which was a chemical dye related to arsenic. Ehrlich was looking for a 'magic bullet' that would selectively attack an infecting organism while leaving the host unharmed. Salvarsan proved helpful to patients with syphilis, but its effect was unreliable and the side effects were often debilitating.[2]

Penicillin Discovered

The discovery of penicillin by Alexander Fleming in 1928 marked a turning point in medicine—arguably, the most important in all of medicine. Fleming noticed a clear zone around a colony of *Staphylococcus aureus* that had been planted on an agar plate. On closer examination, he saw that a spore of the mold *Penicillium* had fallen on the plate, killing the bacteria close to it. But despite his findings, the matter was not investigated further until more than 10 years later. Two Oxford University researchers, Howard Florey and Ernst Chain, produced a *Penicillium* sample and tested it on mice that had been injected with streptococci. Mice that were inoculated with the *Penicillium* survived; the untreated mice died. Fleming called the agent 'penicillin' after the mold that produced it.

The production and purification of penicillin was a long and laborious process, which produced only small amounts of the drug. It was used mainly by the military during World War II and was credited with curing pneumonia, bacteremia, and gangrene, and with saving the lives of many soldiers. But the public was not generally aware of penicillin until victims of the Coconut Grove nightclub fire in Boston were successfully treated with the new drug to combat infection in burn sites. The media proclaimed penicillin a 'miracle drug,' and renewed interest spurred further development and production of the antibiotic. Penicillin became available to the public in 1944 as an over-the-counter medication. It was safe and had fewer side effects than the sulfonamides, except for rare allergic reactions.

Penicillin appeared in an array of products, and soon indiscriminate use began the spiral of antimicrobial resistance. Penicillin-resistant bacteria emerged and proliferated. Only 4 years after its introduction in 1942, 14% of the *S aureus* strains isolated in US hospitals were penicillin resistant. A year later, that figure rose to 38%. The following year, it was 59%.[1] It wasn't until the mid-1950s that a prescription was needed to buy penicillin. Over the next 30 years, researchers worked to produce penicillin derivatives to combat specific bacteria and to circumvent growing antibiotic resistance.

Classification of Penicillins

Penicillins, natural and semisynthetic, are generally bactericidal by interfering with bacterial cell wall synthesis.[4] The chemical structure of penicillin includes a β-lactam ring, which blocks the bacteria's enzyme, transpeptidase, by covalently bonding with the functional end of the enzyme.[5] Penicillins are especially effective against gram-positive microbes. In addition to the original natural penicillins—penicillin VK, penicillin G aqueous, penicillin G procaine, and penicillin G benzathine—investigators added four additional classes.

The penicillinase-resistant semisynthetic penicillins prevent the penicillinase enzyme in the bacteria from causing resistance to the antibiotic. This group includes cloxacillin, dicloxacillin, nafcillin, oxacillin, and methicillin. Penicillinase-resistant drugs were successfully used to treat staphylococci until methicillin-resistant *S aureus* (MRSA) emerged in the 1980s.

The aminopenicillins include amoxicillin (Amoxil®), ampicillin (Omnipen®), and bacampicillin (Spectrobid®). This was the first group of penicillins to be effective against gram-negative bacteria. The extended-spectrum penicillins were introduced to provide a broader spectrum of antibacterial activity when *P aeruginosa* began to appear more frequently, and when resistant gram-negative bacilli increased, especially among hospitalized patients. This group includes the carboxypenicillins (carbenicillin [Geocillin®, Geopen®], ticarcillin [Ticar®]), as well as the newer acylaminopenicillins (azlocillin, mezlocillin [Mezlin®], and piperacillin [Pipracil®]).

The final group of penicillins, the β-lactamase inhibitors, are combination drugs of a penicillin coupled with an inhibitor. The function of the inhibitor component is to bind to the β-lactamase enzyme to block it while the antibiotic portion of the drug can work without being degraded. This group includes combinations of amoxicillin and clavulanate potassium (Augmentin®); ampicillin and sulbactam (Unasyn®); ticarcillin and potassium clavulanate (Timentin®); and piperacillin and tazobactam (Zosyn®).

Other Early Antibiotics

Between the initial discovery of penicillin and its eventual release to the public, Gerhard Domagk worked with different chemical dyes, seeking antimicrobial properties. Domagk performed in vitro and in vivo experiments. He discovered that Prontosil, a new dye, cured streptococcal diseases when injected into mice. Domagk's test-tube studies failed to produce positive results, but his experiments with the mice were a success. Prontosil was the first sulfonamide. Sulfonamide derivatives followed later, including sulfamethoxazole (Gantanol®, Urobak®), sulfisoxazole (Gantrisin®), and sulfamethizole (Urobiotic®). Unlike the earlier antimicrobials, pyocyanase and salvarsan, Prontosil was nontoxic and could be administered to humans.

In 1939, while studying soil samples, René J. Dubois isolated a *Bacillus brevis* bacterium that excreted a substance that killed staphylococci in a culture. He called it 'gramicidin' because it appeared to kill only gram-positive microbes. The drug proved useful only as a topical treatment for minor skin infections, because it was toxic when given intravenously.

In 1941, American soil microbiologist Selman Waksman was credited with proposing the term 'antibiotic' for naturally occurring antibacterial agents. Today, *antibiotic* is generally used for synthetically manufactured and naturally occurring agents and is used interchangeably with *antimicrobials*.

Aminoglycosides

Waksman continued to look for microorganisms in soil that would show promise as antibiotics. He found a member of the actinomycetes family, *Streptomyces griseus*, which proved to be effective against bacteria that caused urinary tract infections (UTIs), meningitis, and tularemia.

It was also the first antibiotic to be effective against *Mycobacterium tuberculosis*, the bacterium that causes tuberculosis (TB). The antibiotic was named streptomycin. It was the first of the class of aminoglycosides, antibiotics that bind to part of the bacterial ribosome and inhibit protein synthesis.

The initial excitement at finding a drug to combat TB was tempered by the toxicities associated with streptomycin. The drug was ototoxic and nephrotoxic, and resistance developed rapidly. Other agents have been developed over the years to treat TB, including ethambutol (Myambutol®), cycloserine (Seromycin®), ethionamide (Trecator®-SC), capreomycin (Capastat®), isoniazid (Nydrazid®), pyrazinamide, rifampin (Rifadin®, Rimactane®), rifapentine (Priftin®), rifabutin (Mycobutin®), para-aminosalicylic acid (PAS or PASA), and a combination of rifampin, isoniazid, and pyrazinamide (Rifater®). More recently, quinolones have been used to treat this infection. However, similar to the other organisms, resistance to antituberculosis medications has steadily increased.

Neomycin (Mycifradin®), another member of the aminoglycoside family of antibiotics, proved too toxic for general systemic use but became a commonly used antibacterial ointment. Over the next 30 years, injectable aminoglycosides were developed, including kanamycin (Kantrex®), gentamicin (Garamycin®, Gentamar, G-Myticin), tobramycin (Nebcin®, Tobrex®), and amikacin (Amikin®). Netilmicin and paromomycin are also aminoglycosides.

Bacitracin (Neosporin®), which was developed from a *Bacillus* in 1943, is a polypeptide antibiotic that is active against gram-positive organisms and a few gram-negative bacteria. It also proved too toxic for parenteral use but is a common topical preparation.

Broad-spectrum Antibiotics

In the late 1940s, Yale University microbiologist Paul Burkholder made a breakthrough discovery in a soil sample from Venezuela. He discovered a microorganism that inhibited a wide range of bacteria, both gram-positive and gram-negative. The drug, chloramphenicol (Chloromycetin®), proved to be effective against *Rickettsiae*. It was first used during a typhus epidemic in Bolivia. Only a small amount of the drug was available, but all 22 patients with the disease were cured.[2] It was also effective against the bacterium that causes typhoid fever.

Again, toxic side effects limited the use of this drug. A small percentage of patients developed life-threatening bone marrow suppression, including aplastic anemia. Rarely used in the United States today, it continues to be used in third-world countries for severe diarrhea and pneumonia.

In 1948, Benjamin Duggar of Lederle Laboratories in New York introduced another antibiotic with broad-spectrum activity. Duggar investigated a golden-colored material with antibiotic properties that was produced by an organism now known as *Streptomyces aureofaciens*. The substance was originally called Aureomycin, and it was active against the typhoid bacillus and *Rickettsiae* as well as many other pathogens. But unlike chloramphenicol, it exhibited minimal toxicity. It was the first of the tetracycline family and is now known as chlortetracycline. Over the next 25 years, six more tetracycline derivatives were introduced. A new class of antimicrobials, called glycylcyclines, has been developed. The first glycylcycline, tigecycline (Tygacil™), a derivative of minocycline, recently received Food and Drug Administration (FDA) approval.

Macrolides

Erythromycin was discovered in 1952 in the soil fungus *Streptomyces erythreus*. It was the first of the macrolide class of antibiotics. Erythromycin has a bacteriostatic effect on gram-positive bacteria, with the exception of enterococci, for which it has no activity.[3] In the past, it was often the drug of choice for group A streptococcal and pneumococcal infections, but antimicrobial resistance and side effects have limited its use in recent years. Clarithromycin (Biaxin®) and azithromycin (Zithromax®) are semisynthetic derivatives of erythromycin that benefit from a greater acid stability, which allows the drug to reach a greater concentration in tissues. Additionally, clarithromycin and azithromycin are better tolerated than erythromycin.

Lincomycin (Lincocin®) and clindamycin (Cleocin®) are technically lincosamides but resemble erythromycin's spectrum of activity. Clindamycin is more effective against anaerobic bacteria than erythromycin and is used in combination with other drugs to treat *Toxoplasma* and *Pneumocystis*. While similar to clindamycin, lincomycin is not as well absorbed orally as clindamycin and is not as active.[3]

Telithromycin (Ketek™) is a representative of the new generation of macrolide antibiotics named ketolides. It was introduced in 2004 and is used primarily against respiratory infections.

Cephalosporins

The cephalosporins are a large class of antibiotics first isolated from *Cephalosporium acremonium* in 1948. The cephalosporins contain a β-lactam ring like the penicillins and are similar to penicillins. They are also subject to β-lactamase degradation. Once the nucleus of cephalosporin was identified, semisynthetic derivatives were developed and the result is four generations of cephalosporins (Table 1-1).

Vancomycin

In the early 1950s, Edmund Kornfeld, a chemist at the Eli Lilly Company, continued the search for new bacteria by studying soil samples from around the world. One of his contacts was a missionary in Borneo who sent soil samples to Kornfeld. Among the samples, Kornfeld found an interesting new species of *Streptomyces*. He named it *Streptomyces orientalis*. The sample proved difficult to purify, and the antibiotic, which was labeled vancomycin (Vancocin®), was not soluble. The molecule was too large to be distributed effectively by oral administration, and the drug caused pain when it was given by injection.

When new soil samples from India revealed better *S orientalis* organisms, the researchers abandoned their ear-

Table 1-1: The Cephalosporins

1st Generation
Cefadroxil (Duricef®)

Cefazolin (Ancef®, Kefzol®)

Cephalexin (Keflex®)

Cephalothin (Keflin®)

Cephapirin (Cefadyl®)

Cephradine (Velosef®)

2nd Generation
Cefaclor (Ceclor®)

Cefamandole (Mandol®)

Cefmetazole (Zefazone®)

Cefonicid (Monocid®)

Cefotetan (Cefotan®)

Cefoxitin (Mefoxin®)

Cefprozil (Cefzil®)

Cefuroxime (Ceftin®)

Loracarbef (Lorabid®)

3rd Generation
Cefdinir (Omnicef®)

Cefixime (Suprax®)*

Cefoperazone (Cefobid®)

Cefotaxime (Claforan®)

Ceftazidime (Ceptaz®, Fortaz®, Tazidime®)

Ceftibuten (Cedax®)

Ceftizoxime (Cefizox®)

Ceftriaxone (Rocephin®)

Cefpodoxime (Vantin®)

4th Generation
Cefepime (Maxipime®)

*Suprax was withdrawn from the market in 2002.

lier findings and started testing from scratch. The newer vancomycin was still not ideal. To minimize discomfort, it could only be given as a slow, intravenous drip, and it had to be given four times a day. But vancomycin was active against all gram-positive bacteria and offered an alternative to penicillin, to which resistant bacteria were on the rise.

Quinolones and Fluoroquinolones
The quinolones, nalidixic acid, and oxolinic acid, are synthetic bactericidal antibiotics that are active only against

Enterobacteriaceae and are used for UTIs. Quinolones preceded the fluoroquinolones, which were made by adding a fluorine atom to the basic quinolone chemical structure. The fluoroquinolones are more effective than quinolones against Enterobacteriaceae and also have activity against *Chlamydia, Mycoplasma, P aeruginosa*, and staphylococci.

The fluoroquinolones gained popularity as frequently prescribed antibiotics, and many derivatives were formulated. As with every antibiotic before it, however, overuse and misuse triggered the development of bacterial strains that were resistant to the class.

Trimethoprim/sulfamethoxazole

The combination of trimethoprim and sulfamethoxazole (Septra®, Bactrim®, Cotrim®) is effective against many gram-positive and gram-negative organisms. Trimethoprim alone is a folate antagonist, which interferes with synthesis of folic acid in the bacterial cell, allowing the sulfamethoxazole to exert its antibiotic activity.

Carbapenems

Meropenem (Merrem®) and imipenem/cilastatin (Primaxin®) are the two members of the carbapenem class of antibiotics developed in the 1980s. Similar to penicillins, they are β-lactam antibiotics that interfere with bacterial cell-wall synthesis. Imipenem is active against most gram-positive, gram-negative, and anaerobic pathogens. Because imipenem alone is degraded in the kidneys and produces a toxic metabolite, cilastatin is added to inhibit the renal enzyme that causes the degradation.

Meropenem resists renal degradation so it does not need to be combined with cilastatin. Ertapenem (Invanz®) is related to the other carbapenems and was introduced in 2001 but does not provide activity against *P aeruginosa*.

Monobactams

Another β-lactam antibiotic, aztreonam (Azactam®), is the sole member of the monobactam class. It is active against aerobic gram-negative microbes but is not effective vs gram-positive or anaerobic organisms.

Miscellaneous Antibiotics

Nitrofurantoin (Macrobid®, Macrodantin®, Furadantin®) and methenamine (Hiprex®, Mandelamine®, Urex®) are antibiotics used for treating or preventing UTIs, for chronic infections, and for reducing recurrent infection.

Metronidazole (Flagyl®, Protostat®) is used primarily to treat protozoan infections and anaerobic-caused infections, particularly in pelvic and intra-abdominal sites.

The Newest Antibiotics

The 1940s, 1950s, and 1960s were the decades of greatest activity in discovery and production of antibiotics. As antibiotic resistance occurred, there was always another drug to take over. The 1970s and 1980s saw a dropping off of new antibiotic research and only nine new antibiotics have been introduced since 1999. Of these, just two represent new classes.

Quinupristin/dalfopristin (Synercid®) is a member of a class called streptogramins. Quinupristin/dalfopristin is a natural antibiotic composed of two streptogramins and is related to virginiamycin, which has been used in animal feed to promote growth.[1] Quinupristin/dalfopristin received FDA approval in 1999, but only to treat vancomycin-resistant *Enterococcus faecium* infections. This agent does not cover *faecalis*.

The oxazolidinones is a new class of entirely synthetic antibiotics. So far, the only member of this class is linezolid (Zyvox®). Linezolid received FDA approval in 2000 for use against vancomycin-resistant *Enterococcus* (VRE) *faecalis*, VRE *faecium*, hospital- and community-acquired *Streptococcus pneumoniae*, and methicillin-susceptible *S aureus* (MSSA).

Daptomycin (Cubicin®) is the first in a class of antimicrobials known as cyclic lipopeptides. It was approved for treatment of serious skin and soft tissue infections and is active against multidrug-resistant gram-positive bacteria such as VRE, methicillin-resistant *S aureus*

Table 1-2: Rapid Development of Resistance to Antibiotics 1940-1999

Agent	Year of FDA Approval	First Reported Resistance
Penicillin	1943	1940
Streptomycin	1947	1947
Tetracycline	1952	1956
Methicillin	1960	1961
Nalidixic acid	1964	1966
Gentamicin	1967	1969
Vancomycin	1972	1987
Cefotaxime	1981	1981 (AmpC β-lactamase) 1983 (ESBL)*
Linezolid	2000	1999

*Extended-spectrum β-lactamase.
From Bush: *ASM News* 2004;70:282-287.

(MRSA), and glycopeptide-intermediate- and resistant *S aureus*.

Antibiotic Resistance—a Growing Concern

Increasing antibiotic resistance is one of the world's most pressing public health problems. Drugs once considered the standard of care to cure common infections and save lives are no longer effective (Table 1-2). The reason is antibiotic-resistant strains of bacteria, and resistance is increasing even against the new generations of antibiotics. In a growing number of cases, bacteria are resistant to multiple drugs, and for some bacteria there now is no effective therapy.

In the July 2004 report, *Bad Bugs, No Drugs*, the Infectious Diseases Society of America (IDSA) states that, "This year, nearly 2 million people in the United States will acquire bacterial infections while in the hospital, and about 90,000 of them will die, according to Center for Disease Control and Prevention (CDC) estimates. More than 70% of the bacteria that cause these infections will be resistant to at least one of the drugs commonly used to fight them."[6]

Factors Contributing to Resistance

Mutations are a natural occurrence in cell replication. When an antibiotic is not administered properly or is prescribed too often, the susceptible strains of bacteria may be killed, but the resistant mutations survive. The surviving bacteria replicate and pass on their resistance genes to their offspring. Subsequently, curing the infection is likely to require a second- or third-line drug, additional health-care costs, and a longer course of therapy.

In some instances, physicians may feel pressured into prescribing an antibiotic 'just to be on the safe side' when a diagnosis is uncertain or when patient follow-up is unlikely. Patients may request the latest antibiotic, which may have broad-spectrum activity, when a narrow-spectrum antibiotic would be effective. Broad-spectrum antibiotics kill a range of bacteria, some of which are normal human flora. Without competition from these harmless bacteria, pathogenic bacteria can proliferate. In some cultures, injectable medication is considered superior to oral formulas, and injectables tend to be broad-spectrum. These situations all encourage selective pressure, favoring survival of the resistant bacteria.

In developing countries, patients may not be able to afford the full course of an antibiotic, only single doses. They take the medicine until they feel better, but the pathogen may not be eradicated, and the surviving bacteria can proliferate. In some countries, antibiotics are available over the counter without a prescription and inappropriate use can occur. Also, if the quality of the drug is not optimal, bacteria can survive and become resistant.

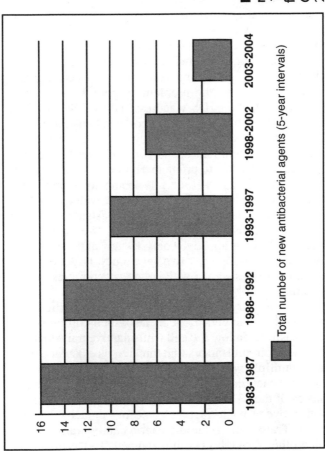

Figure 1-1: Antibacterial agents approved, 1983-2004. Adapted from Spellberg et al, *Clin Infect Dis* 2004;38:1279-1286.

Treatment of animal feed with antibiotics as 'growth promoters' and as prophylaxis for infection is common for livestock and poultry. Researchers have discovered that antibiotic resistance occurs in these animals, and the resistant bacteria can be passed on to humans through consumption of the food.[2]

As a final insult, it is possible for different strains of bacteria that come in contact with each other to share their resistant characteristics, leading to multi-drug resistance (MDR).

Fewer Antibiotics in Development

Pharmaceutical research and development of new antibiotics have greatly diminished in recent years, adding to the urgency of the problem (Figure 1-1). John G. Bartlett, MD, of the IDSA, addressed the US Senate Committee on Health, Education, Labor, and Pensions and the US Senate Committee on the Judiciary in October, 2004, in a plea for government support of incentives for the pharmaceutical industry to promote development of new antibiotics. He said, "Until recently, company R and D [research and development] efforts have provided new drugs in time to treat bacteria that became resistant to older antibiotics. That is no longer the case."[7] The report stated that the FDA has approved only 10 new antibiotics since 1998, and of those, only two have a new target of action and no cross-resistance with previous antibiotics in use.

Plasmids

Bacteria carry supplemental bits of DNA called plasmids within their cells but outside of their chromosomes. The plasmids endow the cell with adaptive traits that help it survive circumstances that threaten its existence. Plasmids multiply within the bacterium and cannot live outside the bacterial cell. They can combine or exchange pieces of their DNA with other plasmids within the cell and between bacteria that come in contact with each other. Traits from related bacteria can be transferred to each other through plasmids dubbed 'F' (fertility) fac-

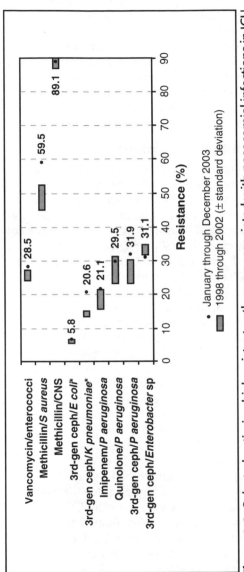

Figure 1-2: Selected antimicrobial-resistant pathogens associated with nosocomial infections in ICU patients, January-December 2003 compared to 1998-2002. CNS = coagulase-negative staphylococci, 3rd-gen ceph = resistance to third-generation cephalosporins (ceftriaxone, cefotaxime, or ceftazidime), quinolone = resistance to ciprofloxacin or ofloxacin.* *Resistance* for *E coli* or *K pneumoniae* is rate of nonsusceptibility of these organisms to 3rd-gen ceph group or aztreonam. From National Nosocomial Infections Surveillance (NNIS) System Report. *Am J Infect Control* 2004;32:470-485.

tors.[2] Genes for antibiotic resistance are often exchanged, and MDR can result.

In 1959, the same four antibiotic resistances were found in two different kinds of bacteria from the same fecal specimen. These plasmids were termed 'R' (resistance) factors. This discovery meant that resistant genes could transfer between unrelated bacterial species, and it opened a new door on the antibiotic resistance problem.

Trends in Antibiotic Resistance

To track trends in antibiotic resistance, surveillance systems have been established that compile databases from participating hospitals and medical facilities. The National Center for Infectious Diseases operates the National Nosocomial Infections Surveillance (NNIS) System, which collects data from more than 300 hospitals, using standardized protocols (Figure 1-2). The CDC also developed the Sentinel Surveillance System, which is used by many states for their data collection. Project ICARE is another CDC surveillance system, which focuses on the epidemiology of antimicrobial resistance in intensive care units (ICUs). Tracking these trends in resistance informs the practitioner of the likely activity of an antibiotic vs a specific pathogen.

Streptococcus pneumoniae. S pneumoniae, a common cause of pneumonia, otitis media, and bacterial meningitis, has become increasingly resistant to penicillin. Data from the Alexander Project, which evaluated community-acquired lower respiratory infections, showed an increase in penicillin resistance in the United States from 16.4% in 1996 to 18.6% in 1997.[8]

The NNIS report and Antimicrobial Use and Resistance (AUR) component indicated highest rates for most antimicrobial-resistant bacteria were found in ICUs, followed by inpatient areas, with the least in outpatient areas.[9] In ICUs, the most common resistant bacteria included MRSA, VRE, quinolone-resistant *P aeruginosa*, and penicillin-resistant pneumococcus.

The Tracking Resistance in the United States Today (TRUST) study, which began monitoring antimicrobial resistance among respiratory pathogens in 1996, analyzed *S pneumoniae*, *Haemophilus influenzae*, and *Moraxella catarrhalis*.[10] The TRUST data for penicillin resistance show an increase from 14.7% from the 1998 to 1999 data to 16.0% for 1999 to 2000.

Penicillin-resistant *S pneumoniae* varied significantly among the nine regions of the United States as designated by the US Bureau of the Census. Resistance was highest in the South Atlantic region (24.8%) and lowest in the New England region (8.3%). When penicillin-resistant and penicillin-intermediate strains were combined, all regions showed greater than 24% nonsusceptibility. The study also stated that resistance was more common in patients 18 years of age and younger.

Data for amoxicillin/clavulanate showed highest prevalence of resistance in the South Atlantic states (22.6%) and lowest in New England (6.7%). Cefuroxime resistance was highest in the South Atlantic states (38.7%) and lowest in New England (18.0%). Ceftriaxone resistance was highest again in the South Atlantic states at 6.7%, and lowest again in New England at 2.0%. Azithromycin resistance was highest in the East South Central states (32.5%) and lowest in New England (15.1%). Erythromycin resistance was highest in South Atlantic states (35.9%), and lowest in New England (17.1%). The East South Central states showed highest clarithromycin resistance (35.8%), and New England was at 17.1%. The South Atlantic was highest in clindamycin resistance at 9.7% and New England lowest at 4.5%. For trimethoprim/sulfamethoxazole (TMP/SMX) resistance, South Atlantic states were high at 40.5% and Mid-Atlantic states were low at 20.1%. Levofloxacin showed the least resistance across the board with a high resistance of 1.0% in West North Central states and a low of 0.1% in New England.

Table 1-3: Rates of Antibiotic Resistance Among *Streptococcus pneumoniae*

Respiratory Antibiotic	Season	% Resistant
Penicillin	1998-1999	14.7
	1999-2000	16.0
Amoxicillin/ clavulanate	1998-1999	10.5
	1999-2000	14.2
Cefuroxime	1998-1999	25.2
	1999-2000	27.4
Ceftriaxone	1998-1999	3.4
	1999-2000	3.8
Erythromycin*	1999-2000	26.6
Azithromycin	1998-1999	22.7
	1999-2000	23.4
Clarithromycin	1998-1999	23.2
	1999-2000	26.3
Clindamycin*	1999-2000	7.2
Levofloxacin	1998-1999	0.6
	1999-2000	0.5
TMP/SMX	1998-1999	27.3
	1999-2000	29.3
Vancomycin	1998-1999	0
	1999-2000	0

* Erythromycin and clindamycin were tested in 1999-2000 only.

Adapted from Regional Trends in Antimicrobial Resistance among Clinical Isolates of *Streptococcus pneumoniae*, *Haemophilus influenzae*, and *Moraxella catarrhalis* in the United States: Results from the TRUST Surveillance Program, 1999-2000.

MDR is a particular challenge to antibiotic treatment for *S pneumoniae*. The TRUST study revealed MDR in 12.2% of the *S pneumoniae* isolates in 1999 to 2000, which was an increase of 11.0% from the 1998-1999 data. Penicillin, ceftriaxone, azithromycin, and TMP/SMX resistance was significantly more common among patients 18 years of age and younger than in older patients, and penicillin, azithromycin, TMP/SMX, and MDR were more common in outpatients than inpatients. In all nine geographic regions, resistance to TMP/SMX was the most prevalent single-drug phenotype, and resistance to penicillin, azithromycin, and TMP/SMX was the most prevalent of the MDR group.

Of nine antibiotics included for the full course of the study, only levofloxacin showed a decrease in resistance, although slight, from 0.6% to 0.5%, from the 1998 to 1999 to the 1999 to 2000 respiratory seasons. Penicillin, amoxicillin/clavulanate, cefuroxime, ceftriaxone, azithromycin, clarithromycin, and TMP/SMX all registered increases in resistance (Table 1-3).

Results from the ARM Program, which is run by the University of Florida, were analyzed for data collected between 1995 and 2003 for *S pneumoniae*, *H influenzae*, *K pneumoniae*, and *P aeruginosa*. The project indicated a 6.5% increase in penicillin-resistance to *S pneumoniae* and a 1.9% increase in resistance to levofloxacin. In fact, antibiotic resistance increased in all four bacterial strains to all antibiotics evaluated, with the exception of decreases found in *S pneumoniae* to ceftriaxone (27.9%) and cefuroxime (14.9%).[11]

The Canadian Bacterial Surveillance Network compiled antibiotic resistance data from 1988 through 2003. Penicillin resistance showed a steady rise until 1998, when a slight drop was recorded over the next 2 years before resistance returned to previous levels.[12] Fluoroquinolone resistance—represented by moxifloxacin (Avelox®), gatifloxacin (Tequin®), and levofloxacin (Levaquin®)—increased, especially between 1999 and 2003, with a peak in 2002. In

2003, resistance levels declined about 0.8% for levofloxacin, about 6.5% for gatifloxacin, and rose minimally for moxifloxacin. Resistance to macrolides has shown steady increases from 1.9% in 1993 to about 15.8% in 2003.

The Prospective Resistant Organism Tracking and Epidemiology for the Ketolide Telithromycin (PROTEKT) surveillance study was initiated in 1999, and the US arm of the study began in 2000. PROTEKT confirmed increasing prevalence of *S pneumoniae* resistance to β-lactams and macrolides.[13] According to the study, although fluoroquinolone resistance is emerging, *S pneumoniae* remains highly susceptible to telithromycin. Clarithromycin also appears to be effective against *S pneumoniae*.[14]

Enterobacteriaceae. Data from 1998 to 2001 for the Surveillance Network (TSN) database-USA, was analyzed for hospitalized patients for in vitro susceptibility to 14 antimicrobial agents for clinical isolates of 10 species of Enterobacteriaceae. The Enterobacteriaceae family includes nearly 80% of the gram-negative bacteria and half of all isolates that are identified in hospitals.[15] The most common isolates are *E coli*, *K pneumoniae*, *Proteus mirabilis*, *Serratia marcescens*, and Enterobacter species.

Except for TMP/SMX, resistance for all Enterobacteriaceae was up to 10% greater in ICU patients than non-ICU patients. Resistance to ampicillin/sulbactam was greater than for any other agent for 9 of the 10 Enterobacteriaceae species in the study, and greater than in previous studies. But *P mirabilis* was more resistant to ciprofloxacin, levofloxacin, and TMP/SMX than to ampicillin/sulbactam. Ticarcillin was the agent with the next highest rate of resistance. Gentamicin was more resistant than amikacin.

The carbapenems had a low resistance rate of 0.001% for all Enterbactericeae tested.

Resistance to fluoroquinolones showed the greatest relative increase of all agents studied, with resistance greater in adults than children. The rising development of resistance to fluoroquinolones may be the result of widespread use of these agents. Fluoroquinolone resistance was also more common as a part of coresistance phenotypes than as a single-agent resistant phenotype. Enterobacteriaceae that were resistant to fluoroquinolones were also often resistant to extended-spectrum cephalosporins, aminoglycosides, and TMP/SMX. Because fluoroquinolone resistance among gram-negative species is evident primarily among MDR isolates, it is likely that fluoroquinolone resistance will be maintained or even increase if other antimicrobials are used. Strains of MDR Enterobacteriaceae have been isolated with increasing frequency in hospitals.

Results from the TRUST surveillance initiative were similar to the TSN study.[16] Levofloxacin proved more active against *P mirabilis* than were either ciprofloxacin or gatifloxacin, but all three agents were equally active against urinary isolates of *E coli*.

The SENTRY Antimicrobial Surveillance Program was launched in 1997. It is a global network for longitudinal tracking of antimicrobial resistance. Significant among its findings were 23 outbreaks or clusters among Enterobacteriaceae that either produced extended-spectrum β-lactamases (ESBLs) or possessed resistance to fluoroquinolones.

Haemophilus influenzae. The Alexander Project 1996-1997 indicated that 30.4% of *H influenzae* were β-lactamase producers in 1996, and 23.3% were in 1997.[8] Results from the ARM Program indicated that resistance to ampicillin increased 11.6% between 1995 and 2003 and 1.3% to ceftriaxone, for *H influenzae*.[11]

Data from the TRUST study did not identify any significant changes in susceptibility between 1998 and 1999 and 1999 and 2000 in the agents tested: TMP/SMX, levofloxacin, clarithromycin, azithromycin, ampicillin, amoxicillin/clavulanate, cefuroxime, and ceftriaxone.[10] TMP/SMX showed the greatest increase, up to 14% in 1999 to 2000 from 11.7% in 1998 to 1999.

The PROTEKT global surveillance study (2000) reported no fluoroquinolone resistance for *H influenzae*, but the prevalence of β-lactamase-producing strains of *H influenzae* was widespread. The macrolides and telithromycin remain generally active.[17]

Moraxella catarrhalis. Study results from the Alexander Project 1996-1997 reported that β-lactamases were among isolates of *M catarrhalis* in more than 90% of the isolates tested.[8]

In the TRUST study, β-lactamases from *M catarrhalis* isolates were similar for the 1998 to 1999 data (93.4%) and the 1999 to 2000 data (94.9%). North American and European studies report rates of β-lactamase production in clinical isolates *of M catarrhalis* to be greater than 90%. Until the late 1970s, *M catarrhalis* isolates did not appear to show evidence of β-lactamases, but now nearly all isolates contain them.[10]

As in the case of *H influenzae*, the PROTEKT surveillance study reported widespread prevalence of β-lactamase-producing *M catarrhalis*, but good susceptibility for fluoroquinolones, macrolides, and telithromycin.[17]

Staphylococcus aureus. In hospitals around the world, *S aureus* is the most common cause of infection. According to the CDC, it affects as many as 9 million Americans yearly.[1] Three features of *S aureus* make it especially threatening: its virulence, its ability to adapt to various environmental conditions, and its ability to cause life-threatening infections.

Methicillin-resistant S aureus *(MRSA).* When penicillin resistance in staphylococci reached alarming heights, the introduction of methicillin in 1959 seemed to be the answer because it was penicillinase resistant. MRSA followed quickly in the early 1960s,[18] however, and the prevalence of MRSA has increased worldwide, first as a nosocomial infection and now in the community.

From March 1995 through September 2002, the Surveillance and Control of Pathogens of Epidemiological Importance (SCOPE) study analyzed trends in the epidemiology and microbiology of nosocomial bloodstream infections (BSIs).[19] *S aureus* isolates were found to cause 20% of the BSIs, second only to coagulase-negative staphylococcus (CoNS) infections (31%). MRSA was detected in 41% of all isolates tested. While CoNS infections were more common in the ICUs, *S aureus* infections were more prevalent in non-ICU wards. However, the proportion of MRSA was significantly higher in ICU patients than in non-ICU patients (44% vs 40%). Notably, the proportion of MRSA isolates increased from 22% in 1995 to 57% in 2001. The rate of resistance to methicillin among *S aureus* isolates was comparable to rates reported in other studies in the United States, but higher than that identified in northern Europe.

Community-acquired methicillin-resistant *S aureus* (CA-MRSA) first appeared in the early 1990s among Australian aboriginals and native Americans in Canada who had little or no hospital exposure before their infections.[20] Since then, CA-MRSA has appeared in clusters in day-care centers, Native American communities, athletic teams, military personnel, men who have sex with men, and prison inmates in several states. CA-MRSA infections frequently recur in individuals and often spread within families and in day-care facilities. CA-MRSA generally begins as a skin or soft tissue infection and may be mistaken for an insect or spider bite.

A study by the Emerging Infections Program in an eight-county metropolitan Atlanta area analyzed laboratory reports of MRSA between 2001 and 2002. It found that the proportion of CA-MRSA infections increased from 4% in 2001 to 8% in 2002. Typically, the CA-MRSA patients were younger than those with hospital-acquired MRSA (37.9 years vs 66.8 years). Most of the CA-MRSA patients (66%) were treated empirically with antibiotics, and 75% of these received β-lactams, which are ineffective against MRSA.

Vancomycin-resistant S aureus. Treatment of *S aureus* has become challenging since the development of resistance, first to penicillin and then to macrolides, tetracy-

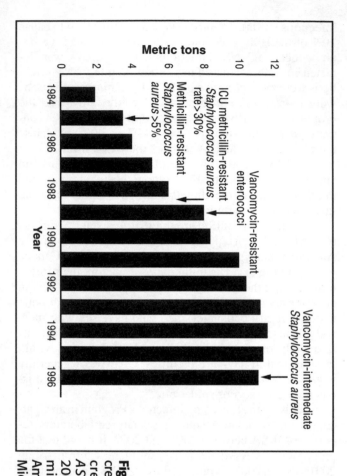

Figure 1-3: Resistance creates markets, use creates resistance. *ASM News*, Jan. 2004. Used with permission from the American Society for Microbiology.

clines, and aminoglycosides. Treatment turned to vancomycin in the 1980s when MRSA became prevalent. The use of oral vancomycin to treat *Clostridium difficile* also increased. This increased use of vancomycin created selective pressure on *S aureus*, which eventually led to vancomycin-resistant *S aureus* (VRSA) strains.[21]

The National Committee for Clinical Laboratory Standards (NCCLS) designates staphylococci requiring concentrations of vancomycin ≤4 μg/mL for growth inhibition as susceptible, 8 μg/mL to 16 μg/mL as intermediate, and those requiring concentrations ≥16 μg/mL as resistant.[22]

The first appearance of vancomycin-intermediate/resistant *S aureus* (VISA) was in 1997 in Japan, closely followed by reports of VISA in the United States, France, the United Kingdom, and Germany[22] (Figure 1-3). VISA appears to develop in patients with preexisting MRSA infections. In the United States, among the few VISA patients studied from cases in Michigan and New Jersey, vancomycin alone has not proved effective.

Surveillance for VISA is hampered by inadequate laboratory methods for detecting the VISA strains. It is suggested that patients with known MRSA infections or those at risk for them be screened. This should include hemodialysis patients and chronic ambulatory peritoneal dialysis patients.

Pseudomonas aeruginosa. P aeruginosa is primarily a nosocomial infection. But once it invades compromised tissue, it can cause serious infections: bacteremia, respiratory infections, endocarditis, meningitis and brain abscesses, external otitis, eye infections, bone and joint infections, urinary and gastrointestinal infections, and skin and wound infections.

Antimicrobial resistance in *P aeruginosa* continues to increase, especially to the fluoroquinolones, cephalosporins, and carbapenems (Figure 1-2). In non-ICU areas, resistance rose against all the antibiotics except cefepime (Maxipime®) and meropenem, for which it dropped

31

slightly.[23] Fluoroquinolone resistance is increasing at a faster rate than resistance to other antibiotics and is a problem both inside and outside ICUs.

Another problem that is slowly increasing is MDR *P aeruginosa*. Tracking MDR rates is complicated by the fact that different studies have used different combinations of antibiotics in their MDR data. In the study reported by Karlowsky et al,[23] MDR was defined as concurrent resistance to any three of the following drugs: ceftazidime (Ceptaz®, Fortaz®, Tazidime®), ciprofloxacin (Cipro®), gentamicin, and imipenem. In this study, MDR was higher than in previous studies: 7.0% to 9.1% in ICU patients and 5.5% to 7.0% in non-ICU inpatients. Rates of all four antibiotics considered in the MDR category showed subtle increases in ICU and non-ICU inpatients over the 1998 to 2001 period.

In a national surveillance study by Obritsch and co-workers of *P aeruginosa* isolates from ICU patients from 1993 to 2002, rates of MDR increased from 4% in 1993 to 14% in 2002.[24] The highest rates of dual resistance were seen for those that included β-lactams and ciprofloxacin; the lowest were for aminoglycosides or fluoroquinolones with piperacillin/tazobactam. The increasing resistance to fluoroquinolones was also verified in a multicenter ICU study (ISS) from 1995 to 2002. This study indicated a 16% increase of *P aeruginosa* resistance to ciprofloxacin during that time.[25]

Data from the ARM Program compiled from 1995 to 2003 showed that resistance to ceftazidime increased 16.2%; to cefepime, 1.5%; to ciprofloxacin, 15.5%, levofloxacin, 2.3%; gentamicin, 16.1%; tobramycin, 10.2%; and imipenem, 10.7%.[11]

Acinetobacter baumannii. Similar to *P aeruginosa*, *A baumannii* is a gram-negative, opportunistic pathogen common in the hospital environment. Hospital-acquired *A baumannii* infections commonly involve the respiratory tract and also include UTIs and wound infections, which may lead to bacteremia. The fact that *A baumannii* tends to persist and spread in the hospital environment makes outbreaks a real threat.

Results from a 1998 to 2001 study that included *A baumannii* antimicrobial susceptibility in hospitals showed increases in resistance to ceftazidime, ciprofloxacin, gentamicin, imipenem, and levofloxacin in ICU and non-ICU areas.[23] Amikacin and cefepime showed decreases in resistance for ICU patients. The only decrease in resistance for non-ICU inpatients was for amikacin. Resistance to the fluoroquinolones was 50%. More than 90% of the isolates were susceptible to imipenem and meropenem, and fewer isolates were susceptible to the other agents. The 2001 rates of MDR for *A baumannii* were higher than those for *P aeruginosa*: 32.5% from non-ICU inpatients and 24.2% in ICU patients.

The SENTRY Antimicrobial Surveillance Program database from 1997 to 1999 indicated that isolates from Latin America were more resistant than isolates from either the United States or Canada.[26] The report stated that carbapenems held the highest activity (90% to 100% susceptible) against *A baumannii* isolates, but also found reports of carbapenem-resistant strains beginning to appear in the literature. As with *P aeruginosa*, the treatment of MDR patients represents a challenge.

Emergence of carbapenem resistance was found in two sequential outbreaks of *A baumannii* in the ICU of a university hospital in Italy between August 1999 and February 2001 and January 2002 to December 2002.[27] And an outbreak of ESBL VEB-1-producing isolates of *A baumannii* in a French hospital was reported as the first such outbreak outside of Southeast Asia.[28]

'Bad Bugs, No Drugs'

In July 2004, the IDSA published a wake-up call regarding a potential crisis in the treatment of antibiotic-resistant bacteria. The paper, *Bad Bugs, No Drugs*, addresses a vital issue in the ongoing war against antibiotic-resistant bacteria. "The pharmaceutical pipeline for new antibiotics is drying up," IDSA president Joseph R. Dalovisio said. "Infectious diseases physicians are alarmed by the prospect that effective antibiotics may not be available to treat seriously ill patients in the near future. There simply aren't enough new drugs in the pharmaceutical pipeline to keep pace with drug-resistant bacterial infections, so called 'superbugs.'[11]

Over the past 30 years, only two new classes of antibiotics have been introduced. The old standard drugs of choice for many infections have been met with resistance from bacteria that can adapt as fast as antibiotics are developed. Of particular importance is the need for development of additional narrow-range agents, because broad-spectrum antibiotics are more likely to spur development of resistance. From penicillin resistance in the 1940s to bacteria resistant to multiple drugs, and most recently, several cases of fully vancomycin-resistant *S aureus*, the trend toward antibiotic resistance continues (Figure 1-2).

The trend toward fewer new antibiotics started more than 10 years ago when half of the US pharmaceutical companies dropped out of the antibiotic research and development (R and D) business or reduced their participation. Of 506 drugs in the development phase today, only five are new antibiotics.[6] Recently, the pharmaceutical and biotech companies have focused their R and D efforts on drugs for chronic illnesses such as cancer, pain and inflammation, metabolic/immunomodulators/endocrine disorders, and pulmonary disease.

R and D for antibiotic development is expensive, time consuming, and risky. According to a recent FDA report, bringing a new drug to market can cost $800 million to $1.7 billion.[6] A report by the Tufts Center for the Study of Drug Development indicated it takes just over 6 years for a new antibiotic or similar drug to pass from clinical testing to FDA review. During this period, the drug's patent, which is usually filed during the pre-clinical phase, is using part of its 20-year life. Although legal, some of the time lost during FDA review is restored, the end result is a shorter patent life for the drug. Additionally, not all drugs make it to the clinical phase of human testing and not all receive final approval.

The federal government has taken some steps to help address the problem of falling antibiotic R and D. In September 2003, the National Institutes of Health (NIH) outlined initiatives to encourage and accelerate research in its Roadmap for Medical Research. In March 2004, the FDA report, *Critical Path*, supported the Roadmap goals by encouraging the creation of new tools to facilitate the drug approval process. Project Bioshield Act was proposed after the 2001 anthrax incidents as an incentive to R and D for new drugs, vaccines, and diagnostics to use against potential bioterrorism attacks. The government would purchase these products. The Bioshield focus is for R and D on smallpox, anthrax, botulism, tularemia, viral hemorrhagic fevers, and plague. Antibiotic development, however, is not included in the Bioshield Act.

The IDSA paper contains recommendations for Congress, the FDA, and the National Institute of Allergy and Infectious Diseases (NIAID) (Table 1-4). Aggressive funding is suggested: double the CDC's antimicrobial resistance program funding to $50 million in 2005 and continue with $25 million increments yearly for a total of $150 million in 2009; increase by $25 million the funding for FDA's programs that support antibiotic development and reduce the cost of clinical trials; increase NIAID's critical translational and antibiotic resistance research efforts; and support synergistic public/private solutions. The paper concludes that "the time for talk has passed—it's time to act."

Economic Impact of Resistance

In addition to increasing the severity of infections, antibiotic resistance is driving up health-care costs. In its paper,

Table 1-4: IDSA Recommendations to Address Antimicrobial Resistance

Recommendations for Congress

1. Provide supplemental intellectual property protections for companies that invest in R and D for priority antibiotics

   a. Establish a 'wild-card patent extension' linked to R and D for antibiotics to treat targeted pathogens

   b. Restore all patent time lost during FDA's review of applications for antibiotics that treat targeted pathogens

   c. Extend market exclusivity for antibiotics that treat targeted pathogens similar to what has been successfully implemented for pediatric and orphan drugs

2. Other potential statutory incentives to spur antibiotic R and D

   a. Provide tax incentives

   b. Provide FDA with additional statutory flexibility to approve antibiotics that treat targeted pathogens as opposed to type of infection and encourage the agency to use that authority

3. Establish similar statutory incentives to spur R and D for rapid diagnostic tests to identify targeted pathogens, which will help to reduce the cost of clinical trials

4. Provide statutory incentives of interest to small biopharmaceutical companies that have far less up-front capital to invest in R and D for antibiotics that treat targeted pathogens

   a. Provide tax incentives to form capital from investors and retained earnings for biopharmaceutical companies that cannot use tax credits, because they have no tax liability, or permit the small company to save or sell its credits

b. Significantly increase the number and amount of Small Business Innovation Research grants that NIH can provide for these antibiotics

c. Waive user fees for supplemental new drug applications submitted to FDA for the treatment of targeted pathogens

5. Provide liability protections to companies that receive FDA approval for antibiotics that treat targeted pathogens

6. Provide limited antitrust exemptions for companies that seek to work together to expedite research on targeted antibiotics

Recommendations for FDA

1. Publish updated guidelines for clinical trials of anti-infectives

2. Encourage imaginative clinical trial designs that lead to a better understanding of drug efficacy against resistant pathogens

3. Provide a clear definition of acceptable surrogate markers as end points for clinical trials of bacterial infections

4. Explore, and when appropriate encourage, the use of animal models of infection, in vitro technologies, and valid microbiologic surrogate markers to reduce the number of efficacy studies required for each additional indication

5. Explore with NIAID all opportunities to streamline antibiotic drug development

6. Grant accelerated approval status for antibiotics that treat targeted pathogens

Table 1-4: IDSA Recommendations to Address Antimicrobial Resistance
(continued)

Recommendations for NIAID

1. Move aggressively to expand the translational research concepts contained in the Roadmap to strengthen antibiotic R and D, remove roadblocks that may exist in NIAID's structure and guidelines, and accelerate antibiotic resistance research activities.

2. Increase the number and size of grants to small businesses, academic institutions, and non-profit organizations that focus on R and D of antibiotics to treat targeted pathogens.

3. Seek greater opportunities to work with pharmaceutical and biotechnology companies to advance antibiotic R and D, and ensure that NIAID staff who oversee technology-transfer efforts understand industry's motivations and goals.

4. Engage more aggressively the infectious diseases research community in research planning efforts and create a more transparent decision-making process.

5. Sufficiently fund and rapidly implement NIAID's newly launched Drug Discovery and Mechanisms of Antimicrobial Resistance Study Section.

Bad Bugs, No Drugs, the IDSA states that the total cost to society of antibiotic resistance is nearly $5 billion annually.[6] The costs of treatment for resistant pathogens affect patients, healthcare organizations, insurers, and society.

6. Encourage research on topics directly related to the implementation of clinical trials.

7. Sponsor research into new rapid diagnostic tests for bacterial infections that, when available, could reduce the cost of clinical trials

8. Re-examine NIH's 1999 research tool guidelines and modify or waive the guidelines where necessary.

9. Develop a fellowship curriculum designed for clinician investigators to provide expertise in clinical trials of new antibiotics.

10. Explore joint programs with FDA to streamline antibiotic drug development similar to programs initiated by NCI and FDA in 2003.

11. Encourage research on antibiotic use patterns and their impact on resistance, specifically the impact of use restrictions on newly approved antibiotics.

12. Fund placebo-controlled trials to determine if certain diseases require antibiotic therapy.

From *Bad Bugs, No Drugs*, IDSA July 2004.

Costs in the Community

When a seemingly simple infection is resistant to first-line antibiotics, the necessarily advanced treatment can double or triple the cost involved, as well as prolong hospitalization. The second- and third-line antibiotics are more expensive and sometimes associated with greater toxicity. Because they may take longer to treat, resistant infections can cause additional lost workdays, extra physician visits, and sometimes, additional laboratory tests. Also, patients colonized or infected with resistant pathogens increase the risk of transmitting them to others.

An example of the cost of antibiotic resistance is the treatment of otitis media, a common childhood ear infection. Because 50% of pneumococci are resistant to routine antibiotic treatment, parents may find themselves back in the physician's office after the initial antibiotic fails. The total cost to the US health-care system from otitis media is estimated at $3 billion to $4 billion yearly, and the impact in Canada is estimated at $600 million per year.[29]

Costs in the Hospital

Every year, about 2 million hospitalized patients acquire bacterial infections while in the hospital, and nearly 70% of those infections are resistant to at least one antibiotic.[6] The number of immunocompromised patients and the quantity of antibiotics administered make hospitals an environment ripe for development of resistant pathogens.

Several studies have pinpointed the costs of MRSA in hospitals. A Duke University Medical Center study of hospital costs caused by MSRA found that the average hospital stay was extended by 4 days if the patient acquired non-resistant *S aureus* vs an additional 12 days for MSRA.[30] The average added cost of the MRSA infections was $27,083, compared to $9,661 for the nonresistant *S aureus* infections.

In Tucson, Arizona, 36 matched pairs of *S aureus* patients with MRSA and patients with methicillin-susceptible *S aureus* (MSSA) were studied. Patients with MRSA were found to have longer hospital stays (15.5 vs 11 days) and longer antibiotic treatment (10 vs 7 days). The median hospital cost for the MRSA patients was $16,575 vs $12,862 for the MSSA patients.[31]

A study at a tertiary-care hospital in Seattle, Washington, compared the cost of hospitalization of patients with MRSA bloodstream infection (BSI) with patients with MSSA BSI. Controls were used for the patient's severity of underlying illness. The results showed that costs were significantly higher per patient-day of hospitalization for MRSA BSI ($5,878) than for MSSA BSI ($2,073).[32] Additionally, patients with MRSA BSI were found to have repeated hospitalizations, compounding the expense of antibiotic resistance.

As antibiotic resistance develops against the latest drugs, the costs will multiply for the discovery, research, and development of new antibiotics and new ways to attack antibiotic-resistant bacteria.

References

1.   Shnayerson M, Plotkin MJ: *The Killers Within*. Boston, MA, Little, Brown and Co, 2002, pp 24, 30, 32, 35-36, 102.

2.   Levy SB: *The Antibiotic Paradox: How the Misuse of Antibiotics Destroys Their Curative Powers*, 2nd ed. Cambridge, MA, Perseus Publishing, 2002, pp 8, 15, 21, 33-36, 47-48, 72-75, 153.

3.   Beers MH, Berkow R, eds: *The Merck Manual*, 17th ed. Whitehouse Station, NJ, Merck Research Laboratories, 1999, pp 1114, 1147-1176.

4.   Jacobs RA, Guglielmo BJ: Anti-infective chemotherapeutic and antibiotic agents. In: Tierney LM Jr, McPhee SJ, Papadakis MA, eds. *Current Medical Diagnosis & Treatment*, 43rd ed. New York, NY, Lange Medical Books/McGraw-Hill, 2004, p 1495.

5.   Musher DM: Diseases caused by gram-positive bacteria. In: Braunwald E, Fauci AS, Kasper DL, et al, eds. *Harrison's Principles of Internal Medicine*, 15th ed. New York, NY, McGraw-Hill, 2001, p 886.

6.   Infectious Diseases Society of America report: *Bad Bugs, No Drugs*. July 2004, pp 3, 14. Available at: http://www.fda.gov/ohrms/dockets/04s0233/04s-0233-c000005-03-IDSA-vol1.pdf. Accessed November 28, 2004.

7.   'Bioshield II' testimony before Senate Committee on Health, Education, Labor, and Pensions October 6, 2004. Presented by John

G. Bartlett, Infectious Diseases Society of America. Available at: http://www.idsociety.org/PrinterTemplate.cfm?Section=Home&Template=/ContentManagement/ContentDisplay.cfm&ContentID=10303. Accessed November 28, 2004.

8.   Felmingham D, Gruneberg RN: The Alexander Project 1996-1997: latest susceptibility data from this international study of bacterial pathogens from community-acquired lower respiratory tract infections. *J Antimicrob Chemother* 2000;45:191-203.

9.   National Nosocomial Infections Surveillance (NNIS) System: National nosocomial infections surveillance (NNIS) system report, data summary from January 1992 through June 2004, issued October 2004. *Am J Infect Control* 2004;32:470-485.

10.   Thornsberry C, Sahm DF, Kelly LJ, et al: Regional trends in antimicrobial resistance among clinical isolates of *Streptococcus pneumoniae, Haemophilis influenzae*, and *Moraxella catarrhalis* in the United States: Results from the TRUST Surveillance Program, 1999-2000. *Clin Infect Dis* 2002;34:S4-S16.

11.   Gums JG: Nosocomial respiratory pathogens: trends in antibiotic resistance, 1995-2003. Results of the Antimicrobial Resistance Management (ARM) Program. *Chest* 2004;126(suppl 4):717S.

12.   Mt. Sinai Hospital, Department of Microbiology. Canadian Bacterial Surveillance Network. Available at http://microbiology.mtsinai.on.ca/data/sp/sp_2003.shtml1#figure1. Accessed December 2, 2004.

13.   Rybak MJ: Increased bacterial resistance: PROTEKT US-an update. *Ann Pharmacother* 2004;38(suppl 9):S8-S13.

14.   Anzueto A, Norris S: Clarithromycin in 2003: sustained efficacy and safety in an era of rising antibiotic resistance. *Int J Antimicrob Agents* 2004;24:1-17.

15.   Karlowsky JA, Jones ME, Thornsberry C, et al: Trends in antimicrobial susceptibilities among Enterobacteriaceae isolated from hospitalized patients in the United States from 1998 to 2001. *Antimicrob Agents Chemother* 2003;47:1672-1680.

16.   Karlowsky JA, Kelly LJ, Thornsberry C, et al: Susceptibility to fluoroquinolones among commonly isolated Gram-negative bacilli in 2000: TRUST and TSN data for the United States. Tracking Resistance in the United States Today. The Surveillance Network. *Int J Antimicrob Agents* 2000;19:21-31.

17.   Hoban D, Felmingham D: The PROTEKT surveillance study: antimicrobial susceptibility of *Haemophilus influenzae* and *Moraxella catarrhalis* from community-acquired respiratory tract infections. *J Antimicrob Chemother* 2002;50(suppl S1):49-59.

18.   Benner EJ, Kayser FH: Growing clinical significance of methicillin-resistant *Staphylococcus aureus*. *Lancet* 1968;2:741.

19.   Wisplinghoff H, Bischoff T, Tallent SM, et al: Nosocomial bloodstream infections in U.S. Hospitals: analysis of 24,179 cases from a prospective nationwide surveillance study. *Clin Infect Dis* 2004;39:309-317.

20.   Udo EE, Pearman JW, Grubb WB: Genetic analysis of community isolates of methicillin-resistant Staphylococcus aureus in Western Australia. *J Hosp Infect* 1993;25:97-108.

21.   Lowy FD: Antimicrobial resistance: the example of *Staphylococcus aureus*. *J Clin Invest* 2003;111:1265-1273.

22.   Tenover FC, Biddle JW, Lancaster MV: Increasing resistance to vancomycin and other glycopeptides in *Staphylococcus aureus*. *Emerg Infect Dis* 2001;7:327-332.

23.   Karlowsky JA, Draghi DC, Jones ME, et al: Surveillance for antimicrobial susceptibility among clinical isolates of *Pseudomonas aeruginosa* and *Acinetobacter baumannii* from hospitalized patients in the United States, 1998 to 2001. *Antimicrob Agents Chemother* 2003;47:1681-1688.

24.   Obritsch MD, Fish DN, Maclaren R, et al: National surveillance of antimicrobial resistance in *Pseudomonas aeruginosa* isolates obtained from intensive care unit patients from 1993 to 2002. *Antimicrob Agents Chemother* 2004;48:4606-4610.

25.   Friedland I, Gallagher G, King T, et al: Antimicrobial susceptibility patterns in *Pseudomonas aeruginosa*: data from a multicenter Intensive Care unit Surveillance Study (ISS) in the United States. *J Chemother* 2004;16:437-441.

26.   Jain R, Danzinger LH: Multidrug-resistant *Acinetobacter* infections: an emerging challenge to clinicians. *Ann Pharmacother* 2004;38:1449-1459.

27.   Zirelli R, Crispino M, Bagattini M, et al: Molecular epidemiology of sequential outbreaks of *Acinetobacter baumannii* in an intensive care unit shows the emergence of carbapenem resistance. *J Clin Microbiol* 2004;42:946-953.

28.   Poirel L, Menuteau O, Agoli N, et al: Outbreak of extended-spectrum beta-lactamase VEB-1-producing isolates of *Acinetobacter baumannii* in a French hospital. *J Clin Microbiol* 2003;41:3542-3547.

29.   Elden LM, Coyte PC: Socioeconomic impact of otitis media in North America. *J Otolaryngol* 1998;27(suppl 2):9-16.

30.   Abramson MA, Sexton DJ: Nosocomial methicillin-resistant and methicillin- susceptible *Staphylococcus aureus* primary bacteremia: at what costs? *Infect Control Hosp Epidemiol* 1999;20:408-411.

31.   Kopp BJ, Nix DE, Armstrong EP: Clinical and economic analysis of methicillin-susceptible and -resistant *Staphylococcus aureus* infections. *Ann Pharmacother* 2004;38:1377-1382.

32.   McHugh CG, Riley LW: Risk factors and costs associated with methicillin-resistant *Staphylococcus aureus* bloodstream infections. *Infect Control Hosp Epidemiol* 2004;25:425-430.

Chapter 2

Penicillin-resistant *Streptococcus pneumoniae*

S treptococcus pneumoniae is the leading cause of community-acquired pneumonia in the United States, as well as of bacterial meningitis and otitis media. It is also a frequent cause of bacteremia.[1] Before antimicrobial therapy was available, mortality was approximately 80% for patients hospitalized with bacteremic pneumococcal infections.[2] Penicillin and other β-lactams became the treatments of choice for these diseases and remained effective for many years. Penicillin-resistant *S pneumoniae* (PRSP) was first described in 1964, and penicillin resistance has continued to climb since then.

Clinical Microbiology

Cell Wall Structure

S pneumoniae is a β-hemolytic, gram-positive, facultative anaerobe. Both gram-positive and gram-negative bacteria have a peptidoglycan cell wall outside the cytoplasmic membrane. In gram-positive bacteria, the peptidoglycan layer comprises repeating disaccharides linked by amino-acid side chains (peptides), forming a thick, meshlike structure. The enzyme transpeptidase initiates the cross-linking of peptides to peptidoglycan. The peptide teichoic acid contains phosphorylcholine, which acts as a docking site for the choline-binding proteins, surface proteins involved in pathogenesis.[3] Other important proteins in the peptidoglycan cell wall include penicillin-bind-

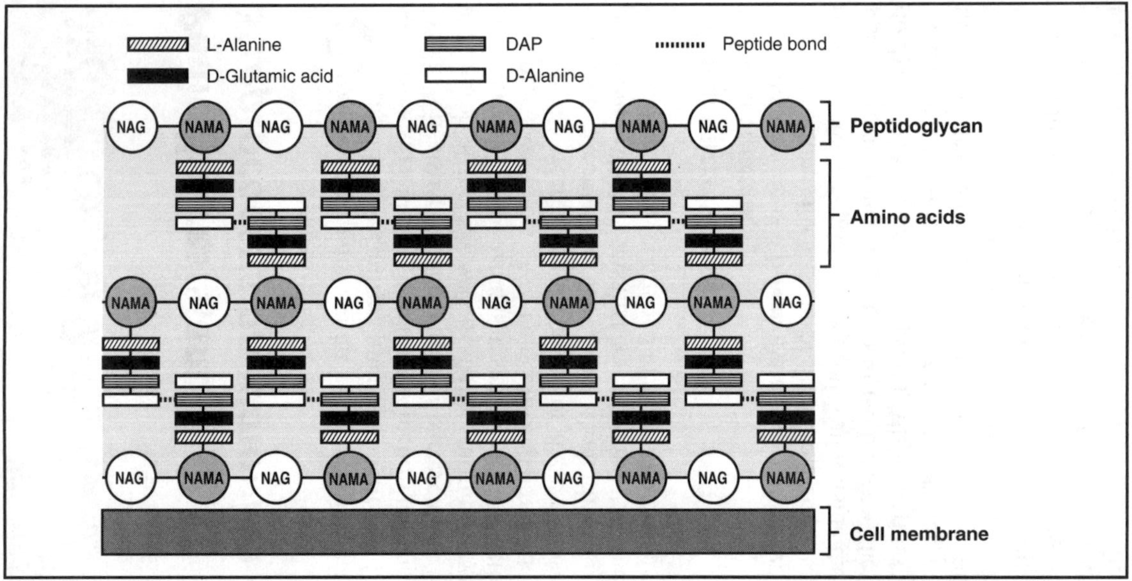

Figure 2-1: The gram-positive cell wall. NAG = N-acetylglucosamine, NAMA = N-acetyl-muramic acid.

ing proteins (PBPs) (Figure 2-1), which are vital to the bactericidal action of penicillins.

Penicillin Activity

Penicillin and other β-lactams inhibit the final stage of cell-wall synthesis in bacteria. Penicillin binds to PBP receptor sites on the bacterial cell and blocks transpeptidase activity. It also removes an inhibitor of the autolytic enzyme, allowing activation of the enzyme, and resulting in cell lysis.[3] Only organisms that are multiplying and therefore actively synthesizing peptidoglycan are susceptible to penicillin.

Penicillin resistance is caused by alterations in the PBPs of the bacterial cell wall.[4] Investigation is ongoing to identify specific PBPs necessary for penicillin resistance. PBPs can be altered by mutations or acquisition of foreign DNA carried by plasmids, bacteriophages, and transposons. Antibiotic resistance can develop rapidly through these mechanisms.

Some bacteria, including S pneumoniae, secrete a polysaccharide capsule that coats the outer wall and affords protection from phagocytosis. Encapsulated S pneumoniae form colonies that look smooth on culture plates and are more virulent than unencapsulated forms, which appear rough on agar plates. More than 90 distinct serotypes have been identified,[5] which makes vaccine development challenging.

Bacterial biofilm is an area of research in antimicrobial resistance. A biofilm is a community of bacteria enclosed in a self-produced polysaccharide and protein matrix that adheres to the environmental surfaces. Biofilms are more resistant to immune clearance mechanisms and to antimicrobial agents than are free-floating cells. Explanations for biofilm resistance to antibiotics include inability of the antibiotic to penetrate the biofilm, transformation of bacteria into a biofilm-specific resistance phenotype with a lower growth rate, and formation of an altered microenvironment.

Pathogenesis and Virulence

Immunity Factors

S pneumoniae is part of the normal nasopharyngeal flora in up to 40% of healthy children and up to 10% of adults.[6] Carriage of pneumococci generally lasts 3 to 6 months, depending on the serotype. Other flora in the nasopharynx may either facilitate colonization through a symbiotic relationship or hinder colonization via competition. Colonizing organisms may elicit an immune response in the host that eliminates the bacteria. The major immune mechanism protecting the host against pneumococcal infection is opsonization, the process by which certain blood serum proteins bind to antigens, altering them for engulfment by phagocytes.[3] Host antibodies react to the bacterial capsular polysaccharides, and C-reactive protein complexes mediate the classic complement pathway to stimulate phagocytosis.

Pathogenicity Process

When the balance between host defenses and bacterial adherence shifts, the four-step process of pathogenesis may begin: adhesion, invasion, inflammation, and shock.[3]

Adhesion. Mucosal pneumococcal colonies alternate between opaque- and transparent-appearing phases. These phases refer to the appearance of the colonies when viewed in cultures, and each has distinctive advantages for survival.

Opaque phenotypes show increased virulence and a greater ability to survive in the blood because of differences in cell-wall proteins.[4] The opaque phenotype also enhances capsular polysaccharide production and pneumococcal surface protein A.

Transparent strains can colonize the nasopharynx more efficiently than opaque strains because of increased teichoic acid and choline-binding protein. Transparent phenotypes also have a greater capacity for adherence to certain cells, including human buccal and lung epithelial cells and vascular endothelial cells.[3] Several cell-surface proteins are active in pneumococcal adhesion.

Invasion. The second step in the pathogenic process is invasion. Once pneumococci infect the lower respiratory tract, pneumococcal pneumonia occurs, and bacteremia may ensue. Of the more than 90 serotypes of pneumococci, only a relatively small number possess enhanced virulence. For example, pneumococcal strains with higher hyaluronidase activity appear to facilitate pneumococcal invasion by degrading connective tissue. The strains are able to cross the blood-brain barrier and have been isolated from patients with meningitis and meningoencephalitis.[3] Another enzyme, neuraminidase, facilitates adhesion by increasing the number of adhesins available for pneumococcal binding.

When the bacterial cell wall undergoes lysis, a cytoplasmic toxin called pneumolysin is released. Pneumolysin damages bronchial and alveolar epithelial cells and pulmonary endothelium. It slows the ciliary beat in the bronchi, which impairs effective clearing of particles. Pneumolysin also causes separation of the tight junctions of alveolar epithelial cells, which allows pneumococci to invade the bloodstream.

Inflammation and Shock. Pneumolysin functions as an inflammatory agent. Pneumolysin is the main inducer of nitric oxide production in macrophages and activates phospholipase in pulmonary artery epithelium. Once activated, phospholipase breaks down cell-membrane phospholipids. This releases free fatty acids, which are cytotoxic and stimulate an inflammatory response in the host. Accumulation of neutrophils causes additional tissue damage and heightened inflammatory responses. β-lactam antibiotics also cause the release of autolysin and subsequent lysis of the cell wall. The generation of cell-wall breakdown products and release of pneumolysin during cell lysis contribute to increased inflammation.

The release of teichoic acid C-polysaccharide during cell-wall breakdown affects activation of the complement cascade. Components of the complement cascade are thought to be essential for generation of the inflammatory reaction in alveoli, meninges, and the middle ear.

Many bacteria have a self-protective system—the two-component signal transduction system—that senses environmental stimuli and appears to contribute to regulation of transformation, autolysis, and adherence.[7] It is thought that oxygen levels, nutrients necessary for cell growth, or peptide concentrations trigger these systems.

Virulence Factors

The polysaccharide capsule of *S pneumoniae* was considered to be the organism's main virulence factor, because bacteria without capsules are largely nonpathogenic. But proteins and enzymes on the pneumococcal cell surface also play specific roles in virulence.[5]

Levels of Resistance

Levels of antibiotic resistance are described according to minimum inhibitory concentration (MIC), which is the lowest concentration of the antibiotic sufficient to inhibit bacterial growth. Penicillin-susceptibility categories determined by the National Committee for Clinical Laboratory Standards range from the susceptible (MIC ≤ 0.06 µg/mL), to penicillin-intermediate (MIC 0.1-1.0 µg/mL), resistant (MIC ≥ 2.0 µg/mL), and high-level resistant (MIC ≥ 8 µg/mL).[8] The rate of resistance, which varies by geographic region in the United States and in other countries, should govern the choice of antibiotic.

Strains of penicillin-intermediate susceptibility were predominant in the United States in the 1980s.[2] Resistant strains emerged, and in 1995 very-high-level resistance was reported in multiple pneumococcal serotypes in three regions of the United States. The proportion of very-high-level resistance to penicillin rose from 0.56% of isolates in 1995 to 0.87% of isolates in 2001.[2] Very-high-level resistant pneumococcal strains are also associated with MDR, a further challenge to treatment.

Epidemiology

Dissemination of *S pneumoniae* is global and increasing. Every year approximately 1 million people become

Table 2-1: **Percentage Penicillin Resistance in the Western Hemisphere, Europe, and the Asia-Pacific Region (1997-1999)**

United States (*n*=4,193)	Canada (*n*=887)	Latin America (*n*=948)	Europe (*n*=1,478)	Asia-Pacific (*n*=746)
14%	6.8%	11.7%	10.4%	17.8%

(From Hoban, et al: *Clin Infect Dis* 2001;52:581-593.)

infected with pneumococci, and the fatality rate exceeds 10%.[5] Particularly alarming is the finding that penicillin-resistant pneumococci are more likely than penicillin-susceptible strains to be concomitantly resistant to other classes of antibiotics.[9]

International travel and commerce contribute (Table 2-1)[10] to the global spread of PRSP and support the suggestion that a key mechanism of transfer of resistance is person-to-person contact. The first penicillin-nonsusceptible pneumococcal isolate of clinical significance (MIC=0.5 µg/mL) was reported in Australia in 1967. By the 1980s, antimicrobial-resistant *S pneumoniae* had become widespread.

In North America, recent surveys have shown a dramatic increase over 10 years in the prevalence of penicillin resistance, from less than 5% before 1989 to more than 50% in 1999.[11,12] Results from the Canadian Respiratory Organism Susceptibility Study (CROSS) of 1997 to 2002 showed increases in both high-level PRSP and multidrug resistance (MDR) in pneumococcal isolates, despite a drop in rates of antibiotic use in Canada.[13] The study found a modest increase in the rate of penicillin-intermediate resistance and penicillin resistance in 5 years and a dramatic increase in the proportion of isolates with high-level resistance (MIC ≥2 µg/mL). This is of particular concern because high-level penicillin-resistant strains are more likely to exhibit resistance to other antimicrobial classes, as well as to other β-lactams.

The first report of infection with a penicillin-nonsusceptible isolate of *S pneumoniae* (MIC=0.25 μg/mL) in the United States was in 1974.

In 1994 to 1995, a national surveillance study involving 30 US medical centers reported a penicillin-resistance rate of 23.6%.[14] The study was repeated in 1997 to 1998 and in 1999 to 2000. Results of the 1999 to 2000 study showed a continued increase in penicillin resistance among *S pneumoniae* isolates in the United States, with a rate of 34.2% PRSP, 21.5% of which were high-level resistant (MICs ≥ 2 μg/mL).[11] The study showed that the proportion of high-level, penicillin-resistant strains exceeded the proportion of penicillin-intermediate resistant strains, rising from 41% in 1997 to 1998 to 63% in 1999 to 2000. Separate studies have identified five major serogroup clones—6, 9, 14, 19, and the most prevalent, 23—of PRSP in the United States.[15,16] Identification of these serogroups is key to future vaccine development.

The ongoing Tracking Resistance in the United States Today (TRUST) study began surveillance of respiratory pathogens in 1996 at national and regional levels. Results from the 1998 to 1999 and 1999 to 2000 studies indicated resistance rates rose from 14.7% to 16.0% for PRSP and dropped slightly for penicillin-intermediate resistant pneumococcal isolates (18.4% to 18.1%) nationally. Regional variations were apparent among the nine regions covered in the study as defined by the US Bureau of the Census. By region, the 1997 to 1998 and 1999 to 2000 data showed similar results, with the highest penicillin-resistance rates in the East South-Central states and South Atlantic region, and the lowest rates in the Mid-Atlantic and New England regions[17] (Figure 2-2).

The Active Bacterial Core Surveillance program, a cooperative population-based study between the Centers

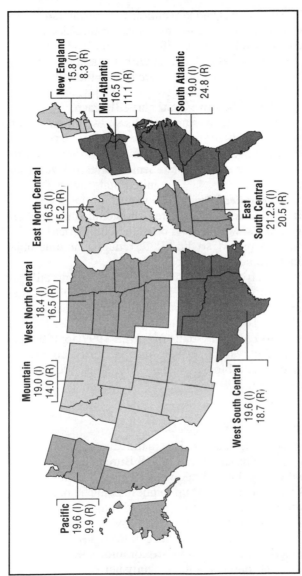

Figure 2-2: PRSP results for pneumococcal isolates in each of the nine US Bureau of the Census regions for the 1999-2000 season. I = intermediate; R = resistant.

New England
15.8 (I)
8.3 (R)

Mid-Atlantic
16.5 (I)
11.1 (R)

South Atlantic
19.0 (I)
24.8 (R)

East North Central
16.5 (I)
15.2 (R)

East South Central
21.2.5 (I)
20.5 (R)

West North Central
18.4 (I)
16.5 (R)

Mountain
19.0 (I)
14.0 (R)

West South Central
19.6 (I)
18.7 (R)

Pacific
19.6 (I)
9.9 (R)

for Disease Control and Prevention and several state health departments, monitored pneumococcal infections in select counties in Oregon, California, Minnesota, Connecticut, New York, Maryland, Tennessee, and Georgia.[9] It also found regional variations, with the highest PRSP rates in Tennessee (35%) and Georgia (33%). California and New York had the lowest rates, at 15% each.

Although different study results show somewhat different rates of PRSP caused by regional variations and differences in study methods, the trend of increased resistance and the number of strains with high-level resistance continues.

Multiple Drug Resistance

MDR pneumococcal isolates (resistant to three or more antimicrobials) were first reported in South Africa in 1977. As PRSP increased, so did MDR, reducing antimicrobial treatment choices for effective therapy.

Analyses from the Active Bacterial Core Surveillance program showed that the proportion of MDR isolates among patients with invasive pneumococcal disease rose from 9% to 14% between 1995 and 1998.[9] The TRUST study analyzed MDR data from the 1997 to 1998 and 1998 to 1999 respiratory seasons, primarily from respiratory tract and blood isolates. That study recorded an increase from 5.9% to 11% in MDR among pneumococcal isolates.[17]

Clinical Infections

As mentioned earlier, S pneumoniae colonizes the nasopharynx in up to 10% of healthy adults and up to 40% of healthy children.[6] Pneumococci may persist for 2 to 4 weeks and can even last up to 6 months. The bacteria are transmitted from person to person through close contact. Therefore, poor ventilation and crowded conditions facilitate the spread of pneumococci. Both day-care centers and long-term care facilities are common sites for S pneumoniae, and outbreaks have also been reported in pris-

Table 2-2: Factors Associated With Penicillin-resistant Pneumococcal Disease

Age
- Children younger than 5 years
- People older than 65 years

Immunocompromised condition
- HIV infection
- Cancer
- Immunosuppression caused by glucocorticoids

Underlying illness
- Cirrhosis of the liver
- Diabetes mellitus
- Alcoholism
- Malnutrition
- Renal insufficiency
- Sickle-cell disease

Respiratory infection
- Influenza
- Air pollution
- Allergies
- Cigarette smoking
- Chronic obstructive pulmonary disease
- Chronic pulmonary inflammation

Environment
- Day-care centers
- Military barracks
- Prisons
- Shelters for the homeless

ons, military barracks, and homeless shelters. Although pneumococci are relatively common pathogens, certain factors predispose patients to infection with penicillin-resistant strains (Table 2-2).

S pneumoniae causes various clinical infections (Table 2-3). There are two basic modes of bacteria transfer to the site of infection: direct spread from the nasopharynx, and spread from the bloodstream. In rare instances, peritoneal infection

Table 2-3: Infections Caused by *S pneumoniae*

Common	Uncommon
• Pneumonia	• Septic arthritis
• Otitis media	• Peritonitis
• Sinusitis	• Endocarditis
• Acute purulent tracheobronchitis	• Pericarditis
• Empyema	• Endometritis
• Meningitis	• Cellulitis
• Primary bacteremia	• Brain abscess
• Osteomyelitis	

can occur from bacteria in the fallopian tubes, and central nervous system infection can arise from a break in the dura.[6]

Bloodstream Infections. Bacteremia may accompany the acute phase of pneumococcal pneumonia, sinusitis, meningitis, endocarditis, or middle ear or mastoid infection.[18] Primary bacteremia—bacteria in the blood without an apparent locus of infection—is uncommon in adults but common in children younger than 2 years.

Endocarditis is caused by bacteremic infection, either from pneumonia or from an occult focus of infection. It may occur in patients with or without previous valvular heart disease, and can cause a new murmur or new valvular lesions. Purulent pericarditis is rare but can occur with endocarditis or as a separate entity.

Bacterial meningitis is most often caused by *S pneumoniae* in adults, toddlers, and infants, except during outbreaks of meningococcal meningitis. Before use of the *Haemophilus influenzae* type B vaccine, *H influenzae* was the leading cause of meningitis in toddlers and infants, and it still predominates in newborn meningitis.[6] Pneumococcal meningitis may be secondary to bacteremia from other sites of infection, or it can arise from a sinus or middle ear infection. Head trauma, dural tear, and cerebrospinal fluid leak also provide entry from infected sites.

Pneumococcal bone and joint infections are uncommon complications of pneumococcal bacteremia. Osteomyelitis in adults caused by *S pneumoniae* tends to occur in the vertebrae.[6] In children, *S pneumoniae* is the causative agent in up to 4% of all bone infections and in up to 20% of bacterial joint infections.[19]

In a report of 42 children with pneumococcal bone and joint infections, 52% experienced either an upper respiratory tract infection or otitis media in the 4 weeks before the documented pneumococcal infection.[19] Once the children were hospitalized, susceptibility data were analyzed from *S pneumoniae* isolates from those who had received antibiotics before hospitalization. Of these cultures, 50% showed decreased susceptibility to penicillin. In addition, 27% of cultures from the children who had not received previous antibiotic therapy showed decreased susceptibility to penicillin.

Intra-abdominal Infections. Pneumococcal peritonitis is rare. It occurs most often in young women and may be related to use of an intrauterine device or to a vaginal infection. A Spanish study of primary pneumococcal peritonitis in patients with liver cirrhosis indicated that hematogenous spread from a respiratory tract infection was likely, with spread from the gastrointestinal tract as a secondary source.[20] The study found a 30.7% rate of PRSP in the 45 cases studied.

Respiratory Tract Infections. Pneumococcal colonization of the nasopharynx is especially common during the winter and spring.[6] The organisms are spread from person to person by airborne droplets and travel along the respiratory tract to the sinuses, middle ear, trachea, bronchi, and lungs.

Pneumococcal infection is a leading cause of bacterial pneumonia. In community-acquired pneumonia, *S pneumoniae* accounts for approximately two thirds of the bacterial isolates.[21] However, although *S pneumoniae* contributes to hospital-acquired cases of pneumonia, the main causes of nosocomial pneumonia are *Pseudomonas aeruginosa*, *Staphylococcus aureus*, *Enterobacter*, *Klebsiella pneumoniae*, and *Escherichia coli*.[22] Empyema is the most common complication of pneumococcal pneumonia, occurring in about 2% of cases.[6]

S pneumoniae and *H influenzae* are the primary infective agents for both otitis media and sinusitis. In the United States, acute otitis media is the most common infection for which antibiotics are prescribed.[6] Although otitis media is usually a disease of infants and children, it can occur at any age.

A 9-year prospective study involving 551 children with acute otitis media found a gradual shift in prevalence of the causative pathogen from *S pneumoniae* to *H influenzae*.[23] Isolates of *S pneumoniae* dropped from 48% in 1995 to 1997 to 31% in 2001 to 2003. In contrast, *H influenzae* began at 38% in 1995 to 1997 and ended at 57% in 2001 to 2003. The study concluded that *H influenzae* had become the predominant pathogen of persistent acute otitis media after widespread use of the pneumococcal vaccine became common. It was also found that fewer acute otitis media isolates were penicillin resistant.

Meningitis and brain abscesses are among the possible complications of acute suppurative otitis media. Hematogenous spread of bacteria may cause meningitis and, rarely, brain abscess as a direct extension of a cranial infection (ie, sinusitis and otitis media).[24]

Acute pneumococcal tracheobronchitis is often a secondary bacterial infection, following an acute viral upper respiratory infection. Again, colonization of the nasopharynx plays a role in the pneumococcal infection.

Skin and Soft Tissue Infections. Cellulitis can arise from *S pneumoniae*, but it is uncommon. Pneumococcal cellulitis is most often associated with immunocompromised patients or those with underlying illness. Complications of pneumococcal cellulitis include bacteremia, tissue necrosis, and suppuration.[25]

Pelvic and gynecologic infections are also uncommon manifestations of *S pneumoniae*. When they do develop, they may occur postpartum or, more commonly, in sexually active young women with multiple partners.[26]

Treatment of PRSP Infections

Penicillin and other β-lactam antibiotics have long been used empirically as first-line treatment for pneumococcal infections. β-Lactam agents are known to have a low incidence of side effects, are relatively inexpensive, and, most importantly, are bactericidal. But bacteria can survive and adapt, giving rise to penicillin resistance among *S pneumoniae* and changing the way pneumococcal infections are treated.

Respiratory Tract Infections. One view of treatment for pneumococcal pneumonia arose from a large, prospective, international study conducted from December 1998 to January 2001.[27] The authors voiced concern that reports of increasing in vitro resistance among pneumococci were causing a shift in the antibiotic prescriptions for community-acquired pneumonia. The shift was from penicillin to the broader-spectrum, higher-potency drugs, such as the quinolones. The fear was that resistance would develop to these antibiotics through selective pressure, making them less useful in the future. The study concluded that β-lactam agents, including penicillin, continue to be effective against penicillin-resistant pneumococcal pneumonia.

New formulations of traditional antibiotics have altered the pharmacokinetics and pharmacodynamics of these agents, which enhances their antimicrobial properties. The duration of antibiotic concentration in serum or tissue above the MIC for pneumococci is key to antibiotic effectiveness. New high-dose and extended-release formulations of traditional antibiotics facilitate such bacteriologic efficiency.

Two amoxicillin/clavulanate formulations were designed to treat respiratory tract infections caused by low-level PRSP (penicillin MIC ≤2 µg/mL). Amoxicillin/clavulanate (Augmentin®) is available as a powder for oral suspension at 90/6.4 mg/kg/d divided every 12 hours. Amoxicillin/clavulanate is also formulated as extended-release tablets, 2,000/125 mg. The clavulanate portion of the drug also provides coverage for β-lactamase-producing pathogens such as *H influenzae* and *Moraxella catarrhalis*. Only these two forms were designed to treat infections caused by penicillin-resistant pneumococci. The extended-release form can eradicate *S pneumoniae* with amoxicillin MICs up to and including 4 µg/mL, comprising most penicillin-resistant isolates. The tablet has a unique bilayer design with sustained-release amoxicillin on top and the immediate-release form on the bottom.

Data from clinical trials confirm the effectiveness of amoxicillin/clavulanate for respiratory tract infections, including acute bacterial sinusitis, chronic bronchitis, and community-acquired pneumonia. In Spain, amoxicillin/clavulanate 2,000/125 mg for respiratory tract infections caused by *S pneumoniae* was evaluated based on data from 10 clinical studies. The patients had acute bacterial sinusitis, acute exacerbations of chronic bronchitis, or community-acquired pneumonia. Amoxicillin/clavulanate showed success against PRSP in 50 of 52 patients.[28] Combined data from nine studies evaluated in Ohio gave similar efficacy results, with 55 of 56 (98.2%) PRSP patients responding.[29]

Other antibiotics exhibiting effectiveness against PRSP include linezolid (Zyvox®) and moxifloxacin (Avelox®). Linezolid, an oxazolidone, has potent activity against all gram-positive pathogens. In experimental animal models, linezolid has demonstrated efficacy against otitis media, endocarditis, and meningitis.[30] Cross-resistance between linezolid and other antimicrobials has not been demonstrated. The fluoroquinolone moxifloxacin is also effective for PRSP in most patients with severe sinusitis.[31]

Otitis Media. Oral amoxicillin continues to be the drug of choice for empiric treatment of acute otitis media. Treatment has changed, however, from the standard dose of 40 to 50 mg/kg/d divided 3 times daily, to high-dose amoxicillin of 80 to 100 mg/kg/d divided twice daily.[32] The high-dose formulation eradicated a high proportion of penicillin-resistant *S pneumoniae* in a large, noncomparative trial of children with acute otitis media. It is generally well tolerated, and its most common side effects in children are mild gastrointestinal disturbances.[32] The consensus of the Drug-resistant Streptococcus Pneumoniae Therapeutic Working Group was that oral amoxicillin should be the first-line antimicrobial for treating acute otitis media. High-dose amoxicillin/clavulanate is an effective second-line treatment for patients who fail amoxicillin alone or for recurrent or persistent pediatric acute otitis media.[32]

Meningitis. The standard treatment for pneumococcal meningitis has been extended-spectrum cephalosporins alone or in combination with vancomycin (Vancocin®). Tolerance to both cephalosporins and vancomycin has been reported, so treatment is turning to newer antibiotics and combination therapy.

Combination therapy with levofloxacin (Levaquin®) and ceftriaxone (Rocephin®) in experimental animal models showed improved antibacterial efficacy over monotherapy with either antibiotic.[33,34] In the experimental rabbit meningitis model, ceftriaxone was slightly less bactericidal compared with levofloxacin against a penicillin-resistant pneumococcal strain, but was much more efficacious when combined with levofloxacin.[34] The combination of meropenem (Merrem®) and levofloxacin also resulted in improved synergistic action.[35] In experimental pneumococcal meningitis studies, daptomycin (Cubicin®) was superior to the standard vancomycin and ceftriaxone

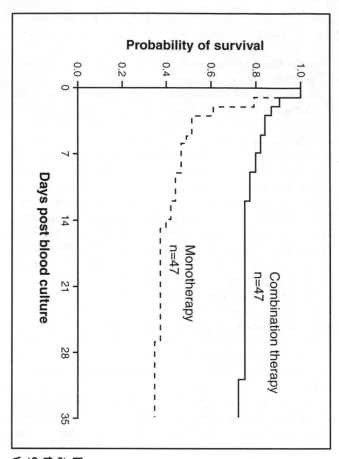

Figure 2-3: Monotherapy vs combination therapy survival plot for 94 critically ill patients with bacteremia.

therapy. It sterilized 9 of 10 samples of cerebrospinal fluid from inflamed meninges.[36]

Bacteremia. Analysis from a prospective, multicenter, international study of bacteremia caused by *S pneumoniae* infection compared monotherapy to combination therapy.[37] β-Lactams were the most commonly prescribed antibiotic. Combination therapies included β-lactam/macrolide, β-lactam/vancomycin, β-lactam/aminoglycoside, vancomycin/other antibiotic, β-lactam/quinolones, double β-lactam therapy, β-lactam/chloramphenicol, β-lactam/trimethoprim/sulfamethoxazole, and clindamycin/quinolones. The results indicated that, although there was no difference between monotherapy and combination therapy for 3-day mortality, combination therapy resulted in lower 14-day mortality for critically ill patients with bacteremic pneumococcal illness (Figure 2-3).

Osteomyelitis. For adults, treatment for PRSP osteomyelitis involves at least 4 to 6 weeks of parenteral therapy.[38] Children with osteomyelitis from penicillin-nonsusceptible pneumococcal strains can be treated with parenteral ceftriaxone or clindamycin (Cleocin®), cefazolin, cefuroxime sodium (Zinacef®), or cefotaxime (Claforan®).[19] Other effective antibiotics for parenteral therapy for children include clindamycin, vancomycin, and cefazolin. Oral therapy is often used as a follow-up to parenteral treatment for children, with clindamycin, amoxicillin (Amoxil®), cefaclor (Ceclor®), and cefprozil (Cefzil®) as choices.

References

1. Centers for Disease Control and Prevention: Assessment of susceptibility testing practices for *Streptococcus pneumoniae*—United States, February 2000. *MMWR Morb Mortal Wkly Rep* 2002;51:392-394.

2. Schrag SJ, McGee L, Whitney CG, et al: Emergence of *Streptococcus pneumoniae* with very-high-level resistance to penicillin. *Antimicrob Agents Chemother* 2004;48:3016-3023.

3. Gillespie SH, Balakrishnan I: Pathogenesis of pneumococcal infection. *J Med Microbiol* 2000;49:1057-1067.

4.   Smith AM, Klugman KP: Alterations in PBP 1A essential for high-level penicillin resistance in *Streptococcus pneumoniae*. *Antimicrob Agents Chemother* 1998;42:1329-1333.

5.   López R: *Streptococcus pneumoniae* and its bacteriophages: one long argument. *Int Microbiol* 2004;7:163-171.

6.   Musher, DM: Pneumococcal infections. In: Braunwald E, Fauci AS, Kasper DL, et al, eds. *Harrison's Principles of Internal Medicine*, 15th ed. New York, NY, McGraw-Hill, 2001, pp 882-889.

7.   Hollingshead SK, Briles DE: *Streptococcus pneumoniae*: new tools for an old pathogen. *Curr Opin Microbiol* 2001;4:71-77.

8.   Kaplan SL, Mason EO Jr, Barson WJ, et al: Three-year multicenter surveillance of systemic pneumococcal infections in children. *Pediatrics* 1998;102:538-545.

9.   Whitney CG, Farley MM, Hadler J, et al: Increasing prevalence of multidrug-resistant *Streptococcus pneumoniae* in the United States. *N Engl J Med* 2000;343:1917-1924.

10.   Hoban DJ, Doern GV, Fluit AC, et al: Worldwide prevalence of antimicrobial resistance in *Streptococcus pneumoniae*, *Haemophilus influenzae*, and *Moraxella catarrhalis*—the SENTRY antimicrobial surveillance program, 1997-1999. *Clin Infect Dis* 2001;32:S81-S93.

11.   Doern GV, Heilmann KP, Huynh HK, et al: Antimicrobial resistance among clinical isolates of *Streptococcus pneumoniae* in the United States during 1999-2000, including a comparison of resistance rates since 1994-1995. *Antimicrob Agents Chemother* 2001;45:1721-1729.

12.   Lovgren M, Spika JS, Talbot JA: Invasive *Streptococcus pneumoniae* infections: serotype distribution and antimicrobial resistance in Canada, 1992-1995. *CMAJ* 1998;158:327-331.

13.   Zhanel GG, Palatnick L, Nichol KA, et al: Antimicrobial resistance in respiratory tract *Streptococcus pneumoniae* isolates: results of the Canadian Respiratory Organism Susceptibility Study, 1997 to 2002. *Antimicrob Agents Chemother* 2003;47:1867-1874.

14.   Doern GV, Brueggemann A, Holley HP Jr, et al: Antimicrobial resistance of *Streptococcus pneumoniae* recovered from outpatients in the United States during the winter months of 1994 to 1995: results of a 30-center national surveillance study. *Antimicrob Agents Chemother* 1996;40:1208-1213.

15.   Corso A, Severina EP, Petruk VF, et al: Molecular characterization of penicillin-resistant *Streptococcus pneumoniae* isolates causing respiratory disease in the United States. *Microb Drug Resist* 1998;4:325-337.

16.   Doern GV, Brueggemann AB, Blocker M, et al: Clonal relationships among high-level penicillin-resistant *Streptococcus pneumoniae* in the United States. *Clin Infect Dis* 1998;27:757-761.

17.   Thornsberry C, Sahm DF, Kelly LJ, et al: Regional trends in antimicrobial resistance among clinical isolates of *Streptococcus pneumoniae, Haemophilus influenzae,* and *Moraxella catarrhalis* in the United States: results from the TRUST surveillance program, 1999-2000. *Clin Infect Dis* 2002;34:S4-S16.

18.   Beers MH, Berkow R, eds: Bacterial diseases. In: *The Merck Manual of Diagnosis and Therapy*, 17th ed. Whitehouse Station, NJ, Merck Research Laboratories, 1999, pp 1147-1209.

19.   Bradley JS, Kaplan SL, Tan TQ, et al: Pediatric pneumococcal bone and joint infections. The Pediatric Multicenter Pneumococcal Surveillance Study Group (PMPSSG). *Pediatrics* 1998;102:1376-1382.

20.   Capdevila O, Pallares R, Grau I, et al: Pneumococcal peritonitis in adult patients: report of 64 cases with special reference to emergence of antibiotic resistance. *Arch Intern Med* 2001;161:1742-1748.

21.   Beers MH, Berkow R, eds: Pneumonia. In: *The Merck Manual of Diagnosis and Therapy*, 17th ed. Whitehouse Station, NJ, Merck Research Laboratories, 1999, pp 601-616.

22.   Chestnutt MS, Prendergast TJ: Common manifestations of lung disease. In: Tierney LM Jr, McPhee SJ, Papadakis MA, eds. *Current Medical Diagnosis and Treatment*, 43rd ed. New York, NY, Lange Medical Books/McGraw-Hill, 2004, pp 212-305.

23.   Casey JR, Pichichero ME: Changes in frequency and pathogens causing acute otitis media in 1995-2003. *Pediatr Infect Dis J* 2004;23:824-828.

24.   Jackler RK, Kaplan MJ: Diseases of the ear. In: Tierney LM Jr, McPhee SJ, Papadakis MA, eds. *Current Medical Diagnosis and Treatment*, 43rd ed. New York, NY, Lange Medical Books/McGraw-Hill, 2004, pp 175-189.

25.   Parada JP, Maslow JN: Clinical syndromes associated with adult pneumococcal cellulitis. *Scand J Infect Dis* 2000;32:133-136.

26.   MacKay HT: Gynecology. In: Tierney LM Jr, McPhee SJ, Papadakis MA, eds. *Current Medical Diagnosis and Treatment*, 43rd ed. New York, NY, Lange Medical Books/McGraw-Hill, 2004, pp 694-727.

27.   Yu VL, Chiou CC, Feldman C, et al: An international prospective study of pneumococcal bacteremia: correlation with in vitro resistance, antibiotics administered, and clinical outcome. *Clin Infect Dis* 2003;37:230-237.

28.   Garau J: Performance in practice: bacteriological efficacy in patients with drug-resistant *S pneumoniae*. *Clin Microbiol Infect* 2004;10:28-35.

29.   File TM Jr, Jacobs MR, Poole MD, et al: Outcome of treatment of respiratory tract infections due to *Streptococcus pneumoniae*, including drug-resistant strains, with pharmacokinetically enhanced amoxycillin/clavulanate. *Int J Antimicrob Agents* 2002;20:235-247.

30.   Xiong YQ, Yeaman MR, Bayer AS: Linezolid: a new antibiotic. *Drugs Today (Barc)* 2000;36:631-639.

31.   Johnson P, Cihon C, Herrington J, et al: Efficacy and tolerability of moxifloxacin in the treatment of acute bacterial sinusitis caused by penicillin-resistant *Streptococcus pneumoniae*: a pooled analysis. *Clin Ther* 2004;26:224-231.

32.   Easton J, Noble S, Perry CM: Amoxicillin/clavulanic acid: a review of its use in the management of paediatric patients with acute otitis media. *Drugs* 2003;63:311-340.

33.   Kühn F, Cottagnoud M, Acosta F, et al: Cefotaxime acts synergistically with levofloxacin in experimental meningitis due to penicillin-resistant pneumococci and prevents selection of levofloxacin-resistant mutants in vitro. *Antimicrob Agents Chemother* 2003;47:2487-2491.

34.   Flatz L, Cottagnoud M, Kühn F, et al: Ceftriaxone acts synergistically with levofloxacin in experimental meningitis and reduces levofloxacin-induced resistance in penicillin-resistant pneumococci. *J Antimicrob Chemother* 2004;53:305-310.

35.   Cottagnoud P, Cottagnoud M, Acosta F, et al: Meropenem prevents levofloxacin-induced resistance in penicillin-resistant pneumococci and acts synergistically with levofloxacin in experimental meningitis. *Eur J Clin Microbiol Infect Dis* 2003;22:656-662.

36.   Cottagnoud P, Pfister M, Acosta F, et al: Daptomycin is highly efficacious against penicillin-resistant and penicillin- and quino-

lone-resistant pneumococci in experimental meningitis. *Antimicrob Agents Chemother* 2004;48:3928-3933.

37.   Baddour LM, Yu VL, Klugman KP, et al: Combination antibiotic therapy lowers mortality among severely ill patients with pneumococcal bacteremia. *Am J Respir Crit Care Med* 2004;170:440-444.

38.   Hellmann DB, Stone JH: Arthritis and musculoskeletal disorders. In: Tierney LM Jr, McPhee SJ, Papadakis MA, eds. *Current Medical Diagnosis and Treatment*, 43rd ed. New York, NY, Lange Medical Books/McGraw-Hill, 2004, pp 778-832.

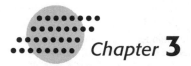 Chapter 3

Methicillin-resistant *Staphylococcus aureus*

*S*taphylococcus aureus* has emerged as a major public health concern because of its virulence and increasing antimicrobial resistance. *S aureus* is the most common cause of skin and soft tissue infections. It can also cause life-threatening infections, including bacteremia, endocarditis, pneumonia, and meningitis.[1]

Penicillin was initially a very effective medication to treat staphylococcal infections. However, once resistance to penicillin emerged, a new antibiotic was needed. Methicillin (Staphcillin®), a semisynthetic penicillin that was impervious to degradation by penicillinase and seemed to adequately address the issue of penicillin-resistant organisms, was introduced in 1959. Methicillin-resistant *S aureus* (MRSA) was first reported in 1961.[2]

Acute interstitial nephritis has been linked to the use of methicillin,[3] and methicillin is no longer commercially available in the United States. Other penicillinase-resistant penicillins, such as nafcillin (Nafcil®, Nallpen®, Unipen®) and oxacillin (Bactocill®, Prostaphlin®), have replaced methicillin in the clinical setting, and oxacillin is used for in vitro susceptibility testing. Nevertheless, the name MRSA is still used for resistant staphylococcal strains.

Today, MRSA is a major cause of health-care associated infections worldwide. Recently, it has also become an important cause of community-acquired infections.[4]

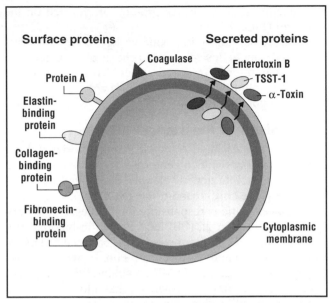

Figure 3-1: Surface and secreted proteins of *Staphylococcus aureus.* Elastin-, collagen-, and fibronectin-binding surface proteins facilitate bacterial adherence to serum components, thereby promoting infection. Enterotoxin B, TSST-1, and α-toxin cause staphylococcal intoxications. Adapted from Lowy, *N Engl J Med* 1998;339:520-532.

Clinical Microbiology

S aureus causes a diverse spectrum of diseases ranging from asymptomatic colonization of skin and mucosal surfaces to invasive and life-threatening infections. *S aureus* is a gram-positive, β-hemolytic, facultative anaerobe that is coagulase positive. Like other gram-positive bacteria, *S aureus* has a rigid peptidoglycan cell wall that is vulnerable to disruption by β-lactam antibiotics, unless the strain is methicillin resistant. Elastin-, collagen-, and fibronectin-binding surface proteins are located on the cell wall (Figure 3-1).

S aureus can thrive in a wide variety of environments and is resistant to desiccation and chemical disinfectants.[1] S aureus is often referred to as 'golden staph' because when it is cultured on sheep's blood agar, the colonies produce a golden pigment.

Mechanisms of Resistance

MRSA strains have emerged through horizontal acquisition of a resistance gene (mecA), which is carried on a larger, mobile genetic element designated staphylococcal cassette chromosome mec (SCCmec).[5]

The mecA gene is responsible for synthesis of penicillin-binding protein 2a (PBP2a).[6] Penicillin-binding proteins are enzymes that are bound to the bacterial cell membrane and act as catalysts for construction of the cross-links of peptidoglycan chains. In MRSA strains, PBP2a replaces other penicillin-binding proteins. It has a low affinity for all β-lactam antibiotics, thus enabling the staphylococci to survive even high concentrations of penicillins, cephalosporins, and carbapenems.[1,6] In addition to the mecA gene, the SCCmec element may contain a series of genes that contribute to antimicrobial resistance, the fem genes (factor essential for methicillin resistance).[6] The fem genes play a role in cross-linking peptidoglycan strands and contribute to the heterogeneity of expression of methicillin resistance. S aureus is considered methicillin resistant when the oxacillin minimum inhibitory concentration is >4 μg/mL.[1]

Pathogenesis and Virulence

S aureus causes two types of syndromes: intoxications and infections. Some species produce exotoxins that can cause food poisoning (gastroenteritis), staphylococcal scalded skin syndrome (SSSS), or toxic shock syndrome (TSS). Evidence suggests that staphylococcal toxins are involved in Kawasaki syndrome and possibly in sudden infant death syndrome and acute exacerbations of atopic eczema.[7] Exotoxins can be produced either in vivo (as in TSS) or in a vector that delivers the toxin to a host (as in staphylococcal food poisoning).

The pathogenesis of staphylococcal intoxications is a relatively simple, four-step process that is regulated by the bacterium relative to environmental conditions. The steps are colonization, bacterial production of toxin, toxin absorption, and intoxication.[1]

The pathogenic process for staphylococcal infections is also regulated by the bacterium in response to environmental conditions but is more complex. Steps to infection include colonization, invasion, adherence to the extracellular matrix, evasion or disabling of host defenses, and destruction of host tissue.[1]

The nares are the primary site of colonization by *S aureus*, but the pharynx, the axillae, the vagina, and damaged skin surfaces may also be colonized.[8] Colonization may be transient or persistent. Persistent colonization increases the likelihood of invasion that results in infection.[8]

Invasion and Adherence

Intact epithelium is generally a barrier to infection with *S aureus*. Once the tissue is broken or a gland or hair follicle becomes plugged, invasion can occur. Adherence is facilitated by protein adhesins designated 'microbial-surface components recognizing adhesive matrix molecules.'[8] These proteins include collagen-binding protein, fibronectin-binding proteins, and fibrinogen-binding proteins. They bind to collagen, elastin, fibrin, fibronectin, and other serum components.

Once anchored to the host tissue, *S aureus* proceeds to disable host defenses and cause damage through the release of toxins, enzymes, and other virulence factors. *S aureus* secretes coagulase, which binds prothrombin, causing fibrinogen to convert to fibrin and possibly shielding the organism from host immune factors as well as antibiotics.[1] The organism also produces membrane-active toxins—hemolysins and leukocidins—that damage red blood cells, neutrophils, macrophages, and platelets. Panton-Valentine leukocidin (PVL), γ-hemolysin, and β-hemolysin create ion-conducting channels in cell membranes that disrupt cell integrity.[1] Exfoliatin, another exotoxin produced by *S aureus,* causes skin erythema and separation, as seen in SSSS.[8] In addition to toxins, *S aureus* produces enzymes—lipase, protease, and hyaluronidase—that destroy tissue and likely facilitate the spread of infection to adjacent tissues.[8]

Evasion of Host Defenses

When staphylococci invade tissue, the host's immune system rallies phagocytes and polymorphonuclear leukocytes to eliminate the organism. In response, the bacteria interfere with the opsonization process, kill phagocytes, and develop methods of survival when engulfed.

Cell-surface protein A interferes with opsonization. Staphylococci that are ingested by phagocytes release catalase, which alters the ability of the phagocytes to destroy them. Bacterial cells can also generate small-colony variants (SCVs). These slow-growing cells are generally resistant to cell-wall-active antibiotics and aminoglycosides, allowing them to resist host defenses and remain alive but dormant.[9]

An especially virulent feature of *S aureus* is its ability to produce superantigens that bind simultaneously to Class II major histocompatibility complex molecules and T-cell receptors. This activates T-cell proliferation that results in a massive release of cytokines, tumor necrosis factor, and interferon. These products in turn cause epithelial destruction, capillary leak, and hypotension.[10]

Pyogenic abscess formation is a hallmark of staphylococcal infection and is another way the organism protects itself from host defenses. The creation of a focus of infection results in a surrounding zone of necrosis. Fibroblasts enter this perimeter area and form collagen, encapsulating the site and impairing leukocyte function and adequate penetration of antibiotics.[1]

Virulence is controlled by global regulatory genes, such as *agr,* which increase the expression of some virulence factors and decrease others, depending on the phase of the pathogenic process. For example, during the early stages of infection, surface-protein binding to the extracellular matrix is important for colonization. After infection is established, the synthesis of exoproteins is essential for the spread of infection to adjacent tissues. The *agr* gene is also involved in development of biofilms. Biofilms develop in two stages: (1) attachment of cells to a surface and (2) cell multiplication and development of a multilayered community.[11]

Epidemiology

MRSA was first reported in the United Kingdom in 1961, and over the next few years isolates were recovered in other European countries, Australia, Japan, the United States,[2] and other parts of the world. By the 1970s, MRSA had become a significant problem in the United States, with documented outbreaks in several tertiary care teaching hospitals. Today, MRSA is a major pathogen worldwide. Increases in MRSA-associated mortality and bacteremia have been reported in England and Wales[12]; in Finland, the number of MRSA infections has risen, with isolates from long-term care facilities accounting for more than half of the MRSA reports in 2001.[13] In Japan, which has the highest rate of nosocomial infections, analysis of *S aureus* isolates collected in a teaching hospital showed an overall MRSA resistance rate of 65.7%.[14] Recently, the prevalence of nosocomial MRSA has risen in Taiwan, Latin America, Malaysia, India, and Australia.[15-19]

The first documented outbreak of MRSA in the United States was reported from Boston City Hospital in 1968.[20] Between 1975 and 1981, nosocomial MRSA became an important pathogen in tertiary care facilities throughout the country. In 1989, a survey of 217 hospitals documented that 96.3% had at least one patient with MRSA and 32% had at least 50 patients.[21] Hospitals involved in the study ranged from community hospitals to large city and university hospitals.

According to the Centers for Disease Control and Prevention (CDC) National Nosocomial Infections Surveillance System (NNIS), MRSA rates in US hospitals increased from 2.4% in 1975 to 29% in 1991, with the highest rates found in intensive care units (ICUs).[22] Other health-care facilities have also recorded increases in MRSA. In 1997, 18% of *S aureus* isolates from a large veterans' home in Wisconsin were methicillin resistant; by 2002, 51% of isolates were resistant.[23] Because antibiotic treatment for *S aureus* had shifted from use of trimethoprim/sulfamethoxazole (Bactrim®, Cotrim®, Septra®, Sulfatrim®) to fluoroquinolones during that period, it was speculated that the increased use of fluoroquinolones might have selected MRSA.

By December 2003, the NNIS reported that MRSA accounted for 59.5% of *S aureus* isolates in ICUs, an increase from 35% in 1995, 50% in 1999, and 53% in 2002 (Figure 1-2).[24]

Nosocomial MRSA

MRSA strains are endemic in many American and European hospitals and account for about one third of all clinical isolates.[25] Within hospitals, the largest concentration of MRSA is found in the ICU (Figure 3-2).[25] Colonized and infected patients are the main reservoir of MRSA in health-care facilities, and the primary means of patient-to-patient transmission is via carriage on the hands of health-care workers. Outside the hospital, long-term care facilities are a major reservoir for MRSA.[26]

Risk Factors

Colonization of the nares with MRSA, either before hospital admission or during the hospital stay, puts the patient at increased risk for development of MRSA infec-

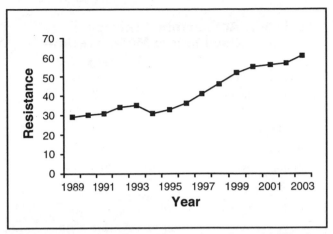

Figure 3-2: Proportion of nosocomial methicillin (oxacillin)-resistant *Staphylococcus aureus* infections among ICU patients, 1989-2003. From the Centers for Disease Control and Prevention: Healthcare-associated MRSA (HA-MRSA). Available at: http://www.cdc.gov/nicdod/hip/aresist/ha_mrsa.htm. Accessed May 23, 2005.

tion. About 20% of the population always carry *S aureus* in their anterior nares, and 60% carry the organism intermittently.[27] Carriage is more common among people with frequent staphylococcal exposure and those with chronic skin disruption. Colonization is higher among health-care workers, dialysis patients, patients with type 1 diabetes, injection drug users, patients with HIV, and patients with chronic dermatologic conditions.[1]

Prior use of antibiotics is an important risk factor in the development of MRSA (Table 3-1). Administration of an antibiotic to which a bacterium is resistant predisposes the patient to colonization by that strain as competitive flora are destroyed and more resistant bacteria take their place.[28]

Table 3-1: Antimicrobial Therapy Used Before MRSA Infection

Antimicrobial Class	MRSA (%) (n = 121)
β-lactam/β-lactamase inhibitor combinations	37.2
Levofloxacin	41.3
Penicillins	6.6
Aminoglycosides	19.0
Macrolides	16.5
1st-generation cephalosporins	40.5
2nd-generation cephalosporins	8.3
3rd-generation cephalosporins	6.6
Vancomycin	24.8
Metronidazole	11.6
Trimethoprim/sulfamethoxazole	10.7
Carbapenems	5.8
All β-lactam antibiotics	67.8

MRSA = methicillin-resistant *Staphylococcus aureus*
Adapted from Graffunder et al, *J Antimicrob Chemother* 2002;49:999-1005.

Previous hospital admission is another risk factor.[25] Furuno et al showed that hospitalized patients who had previous hospitalizations within 1 year of the current admission had a high risk of developing MRSA.[29]

The presence of indwelling devices also predisposes patients to infection with MRSA. These devices create openings in the natural protective barrier of the skin, allowing the bacteria to penetrate. Devices also appear to impair host defenses such as leukocyte function[25] and to enhance bacterial adherence. Additionally, biofilm formation is likely to occur with indwelling devices, creating communities of *S aureus* that are resistant to antimicrobials.[8]

Certain patient populations are at higher risk of MRSA infection, especially those undergoing a surgical procedure. Between 1990 and 1998, about one fourth of liver transplant recipients developed MRSA infection at one transplant center.[30]

Other risk factors for MRSA colonization and infection include advanced age, ICU stay, longer length of stay in the hospital, chronic medical illness, exposure to infected or colonized patients, and open wounds.

Costs of MRSA

Hospitalized patients with MRSA incur greater costs than do patients with methicillin-susceptible *S aureus* (MSSA). One study reported that patients with MRSA tend to have longer lengths of stay (15.5 days vs 11 days) and use of antibiotics (10 days vs 7 days) compared with patients with MSSA infections.[31] The median hospital cost for the MRSA patients was $16,575 vs $12,862 for the MSSA patients. Figures from a study of costs for patients hospitalized with *S aureus* bloodstream infections indicated a median cost of $27,083 for those with MRSA vs $9,661 for those with MSSA.[32]

Preventive Measures

In 2002, the CDC published a set of guidelines for hand hygiene and antisepsis for use in health-care facilities.[33] The document reviews scientific data supporting the need for good hand hygiene, lists recommendations, and suggests performance indicators. Advice is also given regarding use of alcohol-based hand rubs, surgical hand antiseptics, hand lotions or creams, and the wearing of artificial fingernails.

A study of current evidence for the benefits of isolation of hospitalized patients with MRSA concluded that isolation precautions can reduce MRSA even when the organism is endemic.[34] It also concluded that nosocomial transmission of MRSA could be reduced substantially, although evidence was equivocal because different methodologies were used in reporting effectiveness of isolation and confounding factors were mostly lacking.

Community-acquired MRSA

Community-acquired MRSA (CA-MRSA) differs in several ways from nosocomial MRSA. Health-care associated MRSA is likely to be multidrug resistant, but CA-MRSA is usually susceptible to antibiotics other than β-lactams, including clindamycin (Cleocin®), trimethoprim/sulfamethoxazole, and tetracycline.[35,36] Skin and soft tissue MRSA infections are more common among patients with community-acquired infections than among hospitalized patients.[4] Also, most nosocomial strains of MRSA are of SCC*mec* types I, II, or III,[37] while CA-MRSA strains are generally SCC*mec* type IV, and many carry PVL genes.[38]

Since it first emerged as a pathogen in 1990, outbreaks of CA-MRSA have occurred in various populations, including children; Native American communities; prison and jail inmates; high school, college, and professional sports teams; and military trainees.

Athletes who play competitive sports involving body contact and those who share equipment are at risk for acquiring CA-MRSA. Outbreaks in high school, college, and professional football teams have resulted in skin and soft tissue infections associated with turf abrasions and skin breaks, as well as with abrasions caused by body shaving.[39] Use of the therapeutic whirlpool was also a possible source of infection, as was shared equipment and towels. Infection was significantly associated with high-contact player positions.

In 2003, a cluster of MRSA infections was reported among members of a Colorado fencing club and their household contacts.[40] Of the five cases, four involved abscesses, some with multiple sites, and one person required hospitalization for 11 days for paraspinal myositis with bacteremia. The abscesses were located on the abdomen, axillae, legs, thighs, buttocks, and hand and behind the knee. Investigators found that skin rashes were frequent under protective clothing worn by the fencers, and the sensing wire worn to detect a touch by the opponent's weapon was shared and had no regular schedule for cleaning. Additionally, there were no showers in the changing rooms.

An outbreak of CA-MRSA furunculosis in rural Alaska resulted in multiple soft tissue infections.[41] When 34 patients with MRSA were compared to 94 control patients, those with infections had received more courses of antibiotics in the 12 months before the outbreak than had control subjects (4:2) and were likely to have frequented saunas that tested positive for MRSA. In addition, 97% of the CA-MRSA isolates carried the virulent PVL genes.

In 2002, an outbreak of CA-MRSA skin infections occurred at a military base among military trainees.[42] Previous antibiotic use and hospitalization were not factors in the outbreak, but associations were observed between roommates with a prior skin infection or contacts with friends or family who worked in a health-care setting.

An analysis of *S aureus* isolates from children in Southern New England between 1997 and 2001 documented that 40% were CA-MRSA (23 of 57 MRSA cases).[36] Of these, skin and soft tissue infections were common. Spread among family members, frequent use of antibiotics, and child-care center attendance were factors in 35% of cases.

Risk Factors for CA-MRSA

CA-MRSA spread by person-to-person contact is enhanced by previous antimicrobial therapy or hospitalization, serious underlying illness, and intravenous drug use.[25] Skin breaks or abrasions facilitate entry of the organism.

Like other multidrug-resistant bacteria, MRSA is selected for by the administration of antibiotics. In a study of antimicrobial usage and subsequent development of

MRSA, Hill et al demonstrated that the administration of either ciprofloxacin (Cipro®) or a cephalosporin was significantly associated with the acquisition of MRSA.[28] Other studies by Muller et al showed that acquisition of MRSA was significantly associated with use of all antimicrobials and with colonization pressure and that the risk of MRSA acquisition was highest with fluoroquinolones and β-lactam antibiotics.[43]

Clinical Infections

Approximately 30% of adults are colonized with *S aureus* at any one time,[1] and colonization of muscosal epithelium is a major risk factor for *S aureus* infection. The nasopharynx is the primary site for colonization, followed by the axillae, perineum, vagina, and areas of damaged tissue. Skin and soft tissue infections are the most common types of *S aureus* infections, but the bacteria can cause several clinical manifestations (Table 3-2).

S aureus Infections

Intravenous lines or skin lesions are usually the source of *S aureus* bacteremia, but bacteremia may be associated with deep infection, endocarditis, or osteomyelitis.[44] Complications of *S aureus* bacteremia include septic arthritis, osteomyelitis, abscesses of the abdominal viscera or brain, mycotic aneurysm, and meningitis.[1] An analysis of the impact of methicillin resistance on mortality in *S aureus* bacteremia concluded that the mortality rate for MRSA bacteremia is significantly higher than that for MSSA bacteremia.[45]

S aureus is the most common cause of acute bacterial endocarditis[1] and can infect native and prosthetic valves. The signs and symptoms of staphylococcal endocarditis are similar to those of other organisms but may be associated with a more fulminant course. Right-sided endocarditis caused by MRSA is usually associated with injection drug use or venous catheterization.

Table 3-2: Infections Caused by *Staphylococcus aureus*

Invasive Infections

- Bloodstream
  - Bacteremia
  - Endocarditis
  - Mycotic aneurysm
- Intra-abdominal
  - Abscesses
- Respiratory tract
  - Sinusitis
  - Pneumonia
  - Empyema

- Skin and soft tissue
  - Folliculitis
  - Furuncle/carbuncle
  - Impetigo
  - Paronychia
  - Cellulitis
- Musculoskeletal
  - Osteomyelitis
  - Septic arthritis
  - Septic bursitis
  - Pyomyositis

Intoxications

- Toxic shock syndrome
- Scalded skin syndrome
- Food poisoning

Hematogenous spread of *S aureus* can cause abscess formation in the viscera. Infection can also spread from an adjacent deep tissue site. Intra-abdominal organs can be inoculated with MRSA following surgery or penetrating injuries.

Colonization of the nasopharynx facilitates spread of *S aureus* to vulnerable sites. Infection can result from aspiration from the upper respiratory tract or from hematogenous spread.

Staphylococcal pneumonia is an uncommon but serious disease. It may follow endotracheal intubation, prolonged ventilation, or infection with a respiratory virus. Hematogenous seeding can result in lung abscesses, typically by embolization from right-sided endocarditis or from an indwelling venous catheter.[1] Chronic sinusitis and sphenoid sinusitis are also caused by *S aureus*.

S aureus is the most common cause of skin and soft tissue infections.[1] Breaks in the skin allow entry of *S aureus*, leading to infection. Nasal colonization is an important factor. Infection may be caused by direct invasion or a complication of existing lesions.

S aureus infection in or around a hair follicle causes folliculitis, which is often self-limited. If the infection becomes deep-seated and localized, it becomes a furuncle. Furuncles are painful and often cause a fever. When an infection involves a group of contiguous follicles and extends into the subcutaneous tissue, the resulting infection is called a carbuncle. Surrounding and underlying connective tissue becomes inflamed, and bacteremia may develop. Carbuncles are most commonly found on the back of the neck and on the shoulders, hips, and thighs.

Impetigo is a superficial skin disorder that may be caused by *S aureus* or streptococci. Acute paronychia may be caused by *S aureus* and usually requires drainage to aid healing. Burn wound infections are caused by various infectious agents, including *S aureus*. Breast abscess, which may develop during nursing, is commonly caused by *S aureus*.[46]

Direct spread from adjacent infected tissue or blood-borne seeding can result in central nervous system infections. *S aureus* is a major cause of spinal epidural abscess formation, septic intracranial thrombophlebitis, and brain abscess.[1] Spread from infected sinuses may also cause a brain abscess.

S aureus is the most common cause of acute osteomyelitis in adults and a leading cause in children. It is also a major cause of chronic osteomyelitis, which develops at the site of previous surgery, devascularization, or trauma.[1] Prosthetic joints and fixation devices can be sites of staphylococcal infection. Septic arthritis is also commonly caused by *S aureus*.

S aureus urinary tract infections are uncommon but are usually associated with instrumentation or caused by hematogenous seeding.

S aureus Intoxications

Toxins produced by some *S aureus* strains are capable of causing three serious illnesses: TSS, SSSS, and enterotoxin food poisoning.[45]

TSS is an acute, life-threatening intoxication. The most common cause of TSS is the toxin TSST-1. TSS was first described in 1978 following an outbreak associated with tampon use.[1] It occurs infrequently, affecting more women than men. About half of TSS cases occur in menstruating women.[1]

TSS begins with the abrupt onset of high fever, vomiting, and watery diarrhea. A diffuse macular rash is another sign, and sore throat, myalgias, and headache are common. Desquamation, usually of the palms and soles of the feet, occurs 1 to 2 weeks after onset. Hypotension and renal failure are serious complications. Blood cultures are negative for *S aureus* because symptoms are caused by the toxins and not an invasive organism.[45]

SSSS comprises a range of skin diseases caused by exfoliative toxins produced by *S aureus*. Ritter's disease is the most severe form of SSSS and is a syndrome of newborns; in older patients, it is called toxic epidermal necrolysis. Pemphigus neonatorum and bullous impetigo are milder forms of SSSS. At onset, an erythematous rash appears around the eyes and mouth, then spreads to the trunk and limbs. The skin becomes rough or sandpapery to the touch and is tender. Exfoliation begins within a short time, and skin sloughs off in large or small sheets, leaving underlying tissue red and glistening. Large blistered areas may develop, resulting in fluid and electrolyte loss. The course of the illness is usually 10 days. Adults have a higher rate of mortality (50%) than do children (approximately 3%).[1]

Staphylococcal food poisoning is caused by ingestion of food contaminated with staphylococcal toxins. The toxins are often produced in food when it is left at room temperature for prolonged periods. Heat kills the staphylococci but will not destroy the toxins. The symptoms—nausea, vomiting, cramping, abdominal pain, and diarrhea—begin 2 to 6 hours after ingestion of the contaminated food and usually resolve in 8 to 24 hours. Processed meats and custard-filled baked goods are common vectors.

Treatment

There are four basic steps in the treatment of staphylococcal infections: drainage of the infected site, debridement of necrotic tissue, removal of foreign bodies, and administration of antimicrobial agents.

Complete drainage of the infected site is critical in preventing recurrence of infection, as is removal of intravascular catheters, pacemakers, orthopedic hardware, or other foreign bodies at the site of the infection. Vancomycin (Vancocin®) has traditionally been the drug of choice for treating MRSA infections.[7] When patients are intolerant of or allergic to vancomycin, an alternative therapy may be used. Linezolid (Zyvox®), daptomycin (Cubicin®), and quinupristin/dalfopristin (Synercid®) are newer antibiotics that are active against MRSA.

Linezolid

Linezolid is the first member of a new class of antibiotics, the oxazolidinones. Linezolid is approved in the United States and Europe for the treatment of hospital- and community-acquired pneumonia and complicated skin and skin-structure infections. Linezolid has shown consistent activity against almost all gram-positive pathogens, including MRSA.[47]

Oxazolidinones have a novel mode of action. They bind to a portion of the bacterial ribosome, thereby inhibiting initiation of the complex formation for protein synthesis and preventing translation of mRNA.[48] Because this is a unique mechanism of action, linezolid does not exhibit cross-resistance with existing antibacterial agents. Other protein synthesis inhibitors either block peptide elongation or cause misreading of mRNA.[48] Linezolid seems to be especially effective in inhibiting production of virulence factors in staphylococci and streptococci, perhaps because of its mechanism of action. Bacteriostatic activity of linezolid is consistent against gram-positive cocci and is maintained irrespective of resistance to other drugs.

An analysis of two double-blind studies of patients with nosocomial pneumonia caused by MRSA demonstrated that linezolid was associated with significantly higher clinical cure rates and survival rates compared with vancomycin therapy.[49] Linezolid exhibits excellent tissue penetration and 100% oral bioavailability. In pharmacokinetic studies, vancomycin has shown poor penetration into the lungs, which may account for the higher survival rates when linezolid is used. Linezolid is well tolerated orally and intravenously and has been approved in the United States for treatment of nosocomial pneumonia and community-acquired pneumonia. A drawback to linezolid compared to vancomycin is its significantly higher cost.

Myelosuppression, particularly thrombocytopenia, has been associated with linezolid therapy. But studies have shown that linezolid and vancomycin have comparable rates of thrombocytopenia.[50] Additional adverse effects of linezolid include optic and peripheral neuropathy, which persisted in some cases after linezolid was discontinued.[51]

Daptomycin

Daptomycin is the first member of a new class of antibacterial drugs called cyclic lipopeptides. It is active against a broad range of gram-positive pathogens, including MRSA, vancomycin-resistant *Enterococcus*, gly-copeptide intermediately susceptible *S aureus*, coagulase-negative staphylococci, and penicillin-resistant *S pneumoniae*, and it has comparable activity against susceptible strains of these species.[52] Daptomycin is approved for treatment of complicated skin and skin-structure infections. It is administered intravenously.

Daptomycin's unique mechanism of action is the disruption of multiple aspects of plasma membrane function without penetration into the cytoplasm.[53] This mode of action eliminates cross-resistance between daptomycin and other antimicrobials.

Daptomycin's concentration-dependent activity allows for a once-daily regimen and reduces the probability of accumulation-related adverse effects.[54] The adverse-effect profiles of daptomycin and vancomycin are similar for the treatment of complicated skin and skin-structure infections.[55] Daptomycin is generally well tolerated, but reports of myopathy have been documented.[56] Because of the potential for development of rhabdomyolysis, it is recommended that patients receiving daptomycin be monitored for development of muscle pain or weakness and that serum creatine phosphokinase levels be monitored weekly. In addition to the risk of myelopathy, the high cost of daptomycin compared to vancomycin and the lack of an oral formulation are drawbacks.

Quinupristin/dalfopristin

Quinupristin/dalfopristin is a combination of two streptogramins that work synergistically and have a selective spectrum of antibacterial activity, mainly against gram-positive aerobic bacteria. Together, quinupristin and dalfopristin inhibit bacterial protein synthesis; dalfopristin inhibits the early phase of protein synthesis in the bacterial ribosome and quinupristin inhibits the late phase.[57]

Quinupristin/dalfopristin is active against MRSA[58] and is effective in treatment of skin and skin-structure infections and nosocomial pneumonia.[59] Comparative trials have shown that quinupristin/dalfopristin seems to be as effective against skin and skin-structure infections and nosocomial pneumonia as cefazolin (Ancef®, Kefzol®), oxacillin, and vancomycin.[59] Drawbacks to quinupristin/dalfopristin include its high cost and adverse-effect profile (thrombophlebitis, arthralgias, and myalgias).

Some strains of MRSA, especially CA-MRSA, may be susceptible to trimethoprim/sulfamethoxazole and clindamycin.[1] Local antimicrobial susceptibility patterns are helpful in choosing the correct antibiotic for treatment of CA-MRSA. In addition to antibiotic therapy, drainage of infected tissue is an important adjunct to the treatment of MRSA, especially skin and soft tissue infections.

In the last few years, *S aureus* with intermediate resistance to vancomycin has been reported. These strains are termed either vancomycin intermediate-resistant *S aureus* (VISA) or glycopeptide intermediate-resistant *S aureus* (GISA). Combinations of vancomycin and a β-lactam, quinupristin/dalfopristin, or linezolid are recommended for VISA/GISA infections.[1] Recently, fully vancomycin-resistant MRSA strains have been reported.

References

1. Parsonnet J, Deresiewicz RL: Staphylococcal infections. In: Braunwald E, Fauci AS, Kasper DL, et al, eds. *Harrison's Principles of Internal Medicine,* 15th ed. New York, McGraw-Hill, 2001, pp 889-901.

2. Enright MC, Robinson DA, Randle G, et al: The evolutionary history of methicillin-resistant *Staphylococcus aureus* (MRSA). *Proc Natl Acad Sci U S A* 2002;99:7687-7692.

3. Galpin JE, Shinaberger JH, Stanley TM, et al: Acute interstitial nephritis due to methicillin. *Am J Med* 1978;65:756-765.

4. Naimi TS, LeDell KH, Como-Sabetti K, et al: Comparison of community- and health care-associated methicillin-resistant *Staphylococcus aureus* infection. *JAMA* 2003;290:2976-2984.

5. Hiramatsu K, Cui L, Kuroda M, et al: The emergence and evolution of methicillin-resistant *Staphylococcus aureus*. *Trends Microbiol* 2001;9:486-493.

6. Lowy FD: Antimicrobial resistance: the example of *Staphylococcus aureus*. *J Clin Invest* 2003;111:1265-1273.

7. Floret D, Gillet Y, Lina G: Current problems posed by staphylococcal infections in pediatric patients. In French. *Presse Med* 2001;30:1836-1843.

8. Lowy FD: *Staphylococcus aureus* infections. *N Engl J Med* 1998;339:520-532.

9. Proctor RA, Kahl B, von Eiff C, et al: Staphylococcal small colony variants have novel mechanisms for antibiotic resistance. *Clin Infect Dis* 1998;27(suppl 1):S68-S74.

10. Baker MD, Acharya KR: Superantigens: structure-function relationships. *Int J Med Microbiol* 2004;293:529-537.

11. Yarwood JM, Schlievert PM: Quorum sensing in *Staphylococcus* infections. *J Clin Invest* 2003;112:1620-1625.

12. Griffiths C, Lamagni TL, Crowcroft NS, et al: Trends in MRSA in England and Wales: analysis of morbidity and mortality data for 1993-2002. *Health Stat Q* 2004; Spring:15-22.

13. Kerttula AM, Lyytikainen O, Salmenlinna S, et al: Changing epidemiology of methicillin-resistant *Staphylococcus aureus* in Finland. *J Hosp Infect* 2004;58:109-114.

14. Mochizuki T, Okamoto N, Yagishita T, et al: Analysis of antimicrobial drug resistance of *Staphylococcus aureus* strains by WHONET 5: microbiology laboratory database software. *J Nippon Med Sch* 2004;71:345-351.

15. Hsueh PR, Teng LJ, Chen WH, et al: Increasing prevalence of methicillin-resistant *Staphylococcus aureus* causing nosocomial infections at a university hospital in Taiwan from 1986 to 2001. *Antimicrob Agents Chemother* 2004;48:1361-1364.

16. Aires De Sousa M, Miragaia M, Sanches IS, et al: Three-year assessment of methicillin-resistant *Staphylococcus aureus* clones in Latin America from 1996 to 1998. *J Clin Microbiol* 2001;39:2197-2205.

17. Norazah A, Lim VK, Rohani MY, et al: A major methicillin-resistant *Staphylococcus aureus* clone predominates in Malaysian hospitals. *Epidemiol Infect* 2003;130:407-411.

18. Saxena S, Singh K, Talwar V: Methicillin-resistant *Staphylococcus aureus* prevalence in community in the east Delhi area. *Jpn J Infect Dis* 2003;56:54-56.

19. Coombs GW, Nimmo GR, Bell JM, et al: Genetic diversity among community methicillin-resistant *Staphylococcus aureus*

strains causing outpatient infections in Australia. *J Clin Microbiol* 2004;42:4735-4743.

20. Barrett FF, McGehee RF Jr, Finland M: Methicillin-resistant *Staphylococcus aureus* at Boston City Hospital. Bacteriologic and epidemiologic observations. *N Engl J Med* 1968;279:441-448.

21. Boyce JM: Increasing prevalence of methicillin-resistant *Staphylococcus aureus* in the United States. *Infect Control Hosp Epidemiol* 1990;11:639-642.

22. Panlilio AL, Culver DH, Gaynes RP, et al: Methicillin-resistant *Staphylococcus aureus* in U.S. hospitals, 1975-1991. *Infect Control Hosp Epidemiol* 1992;13:582-586.

23. Drinka PJ, Gauerke C, Le D: Antimicrobial use and methicillin-resistant *Staphylococcus aureus* in a large nursing home. *J Am Med Dir Assoc* 2004;5:256-258.

24. National Nosocomial Infections Surveillance System: National Nosocomial Infections Surveillance (NNIS) System Report, data summary from January 1992 through June 2004, issued October 2004. *Am J Infect Control* 2004;32:470-485.

25. Haddadin AS, Fappiano SA, Lipsett PA: Methicillin resistant *Staphylococcus aureus* (MRSA) in the intensive care unit. *Postgrad Med J* 2002;78:385-392.

26. Moreno F, Crisp C, Jorgensen JH, et al: Methicillin-resistant *Staphylococcus aureus* as a community organism. *Clin Infect Dis* 1995;21:1308-1312.

27. Foster TJ: The *Staphylococcus aureus* "superbug." *J Clin Invest* 2004;114:1693-1696.

28. Hill DA, Herford T, Parratt D: Antibiotic usage and methicillin-resistant *Staphylococcus aureus*: an analysis of causality. *J Antimicrob Chemother* 1998;42:676-677.

29. Furuno JP, Harris AD, Wright MO, et al: Prediction rules to identify patients with methicillin-resistant *Staphylococcus aureus* and vancomycin-resistant enterococci upon hospital admission. *Am J Infect Control* 2004;32:436-440.

30. Singh N, Paterson DL, Chang FY, et al: Methicillin-resistant *Staphylococcus aureus*: the other emerging resistant gram-positive coccus among liver transplant recipients. *Clin Infect Dis* 2000;30:322-327.

31. Kopp BJ, Nix DE, Armstrong EP: Clinical and economic analysis of methicillin-susceptible and -resistant *Staphylococcus aureus* infections. *Ann Pharmacother* 2004;38:1377-1382.

32. Abramson MA, Sexton DJ: Nosocomial methicillin-resistant and methicillin-susceptible *Staphylococcus aureus* primary bacteremia: at what costs? *Infect Control Hosp Epidemiol* 1999;20:408-411.

33. Boyce JM, Pittet D, et al: Guideline for Hand Hygiene in Health-Care Settings. Recommendations of the Healthcare Infection Control Practices Advisory Committee and the HICPAC/SHEA/APIC/IDSA Hand Hygiene Task Force. Society for Healthcare Epidemiology of America/Association for Professionals in Infection Control/Infectious Diseases Society of America. *MMWR Recomm Rep* 2002;51(RR-16):1-45.

34. Cooper BS, Stone SP, Kibbler CC, et al: Isolation measures in the hospital management of methicillin resistant *Staphylococcus aureus* (MRSA): systematic review of the literature. *BMJ* 2004;329:533-540.

35. Baba T, Takeuchi F, Kuroda M, et al: Genome and virulence determinants of high virulence community-acquired MRSA. *Lancet* 2002;359:1819-1827.

36. Dietrich DW, Auld DB, Mermel LA: Community-acquired methicillin-resistant *Staphylococcus aureus* in Southern New England children. *Pediatrics* 2004;113:e347-e352.

37. Ito T, Katayama Y, Asada K, et al: Structural comparison of three types of staphylococcal cassette chromosome mec integrated in the chromosome in methicillin-resistant *Staphylococcus aureus*. *Antimicrob Agents Chemother* 2001;45:1323-1336.

38. Vandenesch F, Naimi T, Enright MC, et al: Community-acquired methicillin-resistant *Staphylococcus aureus* carrying Panton-Valentine leukocidin genes: worldwide emergence. *Emerg Infect Dis* 2003;9:978-984.

39. Begier EM, Frenette K, Barrett NL, et al: A high-morbidity outbreak of methicillin-resistant *Staphylococcus aureus* among players on a college football team, facilitated by cosmetic body shaving and turf burns. *Clin Infect Dis* 2004;39:1446-1453.

40. Centers for Disease Control and Prevention: Methicillin-resistant *Staphylococcus aureus* infections among competitive sports participants—Colorado, Indiana, Pennsylvania, and Los Angeles County, 2000-2003. *MMWR Morb Mortal Wkly Rep* 2003;52:793-795.

41. Baggett HC, Hennessy TW, Rudolph K, et al: Community-onset methicillin-resistant *Staphylococcus aureus* associated with

antibiotic use and the cytotoxin Panton-Valentine leukocidin during a furunculosis outbreak in rural Alaska. *J Infect Dis* 2004;189:1565-1573.

42.   Campbell KM, Vaughn AF, Russell KL, et al: Risk factors for community-associated methicillin-resistant *Staphylococcus aureus* infections in an outbreak of disease among military trainees in San Diego, California, in 2002. *J Clin Microbiol* 2004;42:4050-4053.

43.   Muller A, Thouverez M, Talon D, et al: Contribution of antibiotic pressure in the acquisition of methicillin-resistant *Staphylococcus aureus* (MRSA) in a university hospital. In French. *Pathol Biol (Paris)* 2003;51:454-459.

44.   Cosgrove SE, Sakoulas G, Perencevich EN, et al: Comparison of mortality associated with methicillin-resistant and methicillin-susceptible *Staphylococcus aureus* bacteremia: a meta-analysis. *Clin Infect Dis* 2003;36:53-59.

45.   Chambers HF. Infectious diseases: bacterial and chlamydial. In: Tierney LM Jr, McPhee SJ, Papadakis MA, eds. *Current Medical Diagnosis and Treatment,* 43rd ed. New York, Lange Medical Books/McGraw-Hill, 2004, pp 1337-1379.

46.   Giuliano AE. Breast. In: Tierney LM Jr, McPhee SJ, Papadakis MA, eds. *Current Medical Diagnosis and Treatment,* 43rd ed. New York, Lange Medical Books/McGraw-Hill, 2004, pp 669-693.

47.   Gemmell CG: Susceptibility of a variety of clinical isolates to linezolid: a European inter-country comparison. *J Antimicrob Chemother* 2001;48:47-52.

48.   Livermore DM: Linezolid in vitro: mechanism and antibacterial spectrum. *J Antimicrob Chemother* 2003;51(suppl S2):ii9-ii16.

49.   Wunderink RG, Rello J, Cammarata SK, et al: Linezolid vs vancomycin: analysis of two double-blind studies of patients with methicillin-resistant *Staphylococcus aureus* nosocomial pneumonia. *Chest* 2003;124:1789-1797.

50.   Rao N, Ziran BH, Wagener MM, et al: Similar hematologic effects of long-term linezolid and vancomycin therapy in a prospective observational study of patients with orthopedic infections. *Clin Infect Dis* 2004;38:1058-1064.

51.   Frippiat F, Bergiers C, Michel C, et al: Severe bilateral optic neuritis associated with prolonged linezolid therapy. *J Antimicrob Chemother* 2004;53:1114-1115.

52. Tally FP, DeBruin MF: Development of daptomycin for gram-positive infections. *J Antimicrob Chemother* 2000;46:523-526.

53. Alborn WE Jr, Allen NE, Preston DA: Daptomycin disrupts membrane potential in growing *Staphylococcus aureus*. *Antimicrob Agents Chemother* 1991;35:2282-2287.

54. Cha R, Grucz RG Jr, Rybak MJ: Daptomycin dose-effect relationship against resistant gram-positive organisms. *Antimicrob Agents Chemother* 2003;47:1598-1603.

55. Fenton C, Keating GM, Curran MP: Daptomycin. *Drugs* 2004;64:445-455.

56. Veligandla SR, Louie KR, Malesker MA, et al: Muscle pain associated with daptomycin. *Ann Pharmacother* 2004;38:1860-1862.

57. Cocito C, Di Giambattista M, Nyssen E, et al: Inhibition of protein synthesis by streptogramins and related antibiotics. *J Antimicrob Chemother* 1997;39(suppl A):7-13.

58. Bouanchaud DH: In-vitro and in-vivo antibacterial activity of quinupristin/dalfopristin. *J Antimicrob Chemother* 1997;39(suppl A):15-21.

59. Allington DR, Rivey MP: Quinupristin/dalfopristin: a therapeutic review. *Clin Ther* 2001;23:24-44.

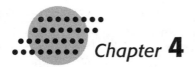

Chapter 4

Vancomycin-resistant Enterococci

Enterococci are part of the normal flora of the human gastrointestinal (GI) tract.[1-4] They are generally considered to be of low virulence, but they can cause serious and life-threatening illness in hospitalized or immunocompromised patients. The urinary tract, bloodstream, and intra-abdominal space are the most common sites of enterococcal infection.[1,2]

Over the past decade, enterococci have become important nosocomial pathogens, primarily because of their intrinsic resistance to many antibiotics and their ability to acquire resistance to most other available antimicrobials.[2,3] Initially, ampicillin was the therapy of choice for enterococcal infections,[4] but as resistance to ampicillin emerged, physicians turned to vancomycin (Vancocin®).

In the late 1980s, vancomycin use increased dramatically in hospitals, mostly to treat the growing prevalence of methicillin-resistant *Staphylococcus aureus* (MRSA) and diarrhea caused by *Clostridium difficile*.[3,4] More than 30 years after vancomycin was clinically introduced, vancomycin-resistant *Enterococcus* (VRE) was detected in England, France, and the United States.[5] In the past decade, reports of VRE have come from many other countries, including Asia, Australia, South America, Africa, and Greece. While the prevalence of VRE continues to increase, effective antimicrobial therapy remains limited, adding urgency to the search for new antibiotics that will treat these pathogens.

Clinical Microbiology

Enterococci are gram-positive, α-hemolytic, group D enteric streptococci. They were originally classified within the *Streptococcus* genus, but were eventually differentiated from nonenterococcal streptococci and placed in their own genus, *Enterococcus*.[3,6] Enterococci are able to grow in 6.5% sodium chloride and in bile, and are opportunistic when epithelial or muscosal barriers are disrupted.[6] At least 17 species of *Enterococcus* have been identified,[7] but most human infections are caused by only two species, *E faecium* and *E faecalis*.[1-3]

Mechanisms of resistance

Intrinsic resistance. Enterococci exhibit intrinsic resistance to a number of classes of antibiotics, including β-lactams, macrolides, aminoglycosides, and trimethoprim/sulfamethoxazole.[7] Resistance or tolerance to β-lactam antibiotics is typical of enterococci,[3,7] and *E faecium* is more resistant than *E faecalis*.[3] The major mechanism of β-lactam resistance in enterococci is attributable to the production of low-affinity penicillin-binding protein (PBP).

Intrinsic resistance to macrolides is caused by altered enterococcal ribosomal targets. Enterococci also exhibit low-level resistance to all aminoglycosides, which cannot efficiently cross the enterococcal cell wall.[7] Trimethoprim/sulfamethoxazole exerts its action by blocking folic acid synthesis, but enterococci are able to extract folinic acid derivatives directly from their environment to bypass this action.[8]

Acquired resistance. Enterococci have the ability to acquire genetic materials that confer antimicrobial resistance. *E faecalis*, in particular, can produce β-lactamase enzymes that impart high-level resistance to imipenem and all penicillins, with the exception of combinations of β-lactam inhibitors with penicillins.[9] Enterococci have also acquired enzymes that inactivate aminoglycosides[10] and other enzymes that modify ribosomal targets.[7,10]

Vancomycin resistance. Vancomycin inhibits cell-wall synthesis by binding to the D-alanyl-D-alanine termini of a pentopeptide cell wall precursor, blocking its addition to the growing peptidoglycan chain and preventing subsequent cross linking of the cell wall.[11] Resistance to vancomycin is mediated by enterococcal enzymes that alter the binding site so that vancomycin is unable to bind to the cell wall.

Five different phenotypes of vancomycin resistance have been described—VanA, VanB, VanC, VanD, and VanE—and others appear to exist.[3,7] VanA and VanB are found primarily in *E faecalis* and *E faecium* and both are transmitted on plasmids or mobile genetic elements.[3,7] The VanA phenotype is predominant in Europe and the United States, but VanB is also fairly common in the United States. VanA enterococci are highly resistant to both vancomycin and teicoplanin (a glycopeptide available in Europe but not in the United States), while VanB isolates are variably resistant to vancomycin and are susceptible to teicoplanin.[7]

Pathogenicity and Virulence

The first step in the infection process is bacterial adherence to host tissue. Because enterococci are commensals in the GI tract, attachment to host cells is crucial to the pathogenic process to prevent elimination of the bacteria through the normal flow of intestinal contents.

Adherence mechanisms

Studies have shown that enterococci can attach to intestinal and urinary tract epithelial cells and to heart cells by means of adhesins.[12] Aggregation substance is an adhesin that is bound to the bacterial cell surface and has a hairlike protrusion. Aggregation substance appears to enhance enterococcal adherence to intestinal and renal epithelial cells and also facilitates exchange of plasmids between *E faecalis* strains, which carry virulence traits and antibiotic-resistance genes. Aggregation substance may also influence phagocytosis.[2]

Table 4-1: Comparison of Known Virulence Factors in *E faecalis* and *E faecium* Species

Factor	Occurrence*	
	E faecalis	*E faecium*
Antibiotic resistance	+	++
Cytolysin	+	-
Aggregation substance	+	Rare
Gelatinase	+	-
Extracellular superoxide	+	-
Extracellular surface protein	+	-

* ++ = most, + = some, - = none
Adapted from Mundy[2]

Carbohydrate adhesins are present in some strains of enterococci. Fibronectin also plays a role in enterococcal adherence by interacting with aggregation substance to mediate adhesion of *E faecalis* to colonic mucosa.[13]

Intravenous (IV) lines, abscesses, and urinary tract infections are identifiable sources of enterococcal bacteremia.[14] Translocation of enterococci from the intestinal tract is another likely route to systemic infection.[1] In the translocation model, epithelial cells or leukocytes in the intestines engulf adherent bacteria, which then migrate in phagocytes to mesenteric lymph nodes, where they proliferate. The bacteria are then carried in the blood to other sites.

Virulence factors

In addition to aggregation substance and adhesins, cytolysin (hemolysin) is another virulence factor and is associated with increased severity of enterococcal infections.[12] Outbreak investigations show that cytolysin occurs in up to 60% of *E faecalis* isolates.[1]

E faecalis has the ability to form biofilm on medical devices such as central venous catheters. The biofilm mass of bacteria increases the risk of catheter-related bloodstream infections.[15] The production of extracellular superoxide, extracellular surface protein (esp), and gelatinase are additional virulence factors that are variable traits of some *E faecalis* strains[2] (Table 4-1). Studies indicate that hyaluronidase may also contribute to enterococcal virulence.[1]

Avoidance or modulation of host defenses is an important step in the pathogenesis process. Studies indicate that enterococcal lipoteichoic acid, pheromones, and peptide inhibitors may act as virulence factors by modulating host inflammatory responses.[1]

Epidemiology

When first detected in 1989, the rate of vancomycin resistance was 0.3% in the United States, as reported in the National Nosocomial Infections Surveillance (NNIS) system report.[16] By 1993, the rate had risen to 7.9%. During that period, VRE infections in patients in intensive-care units (ICUs) rose from 0.4% to 13.6%, a 34-fold increase. Increases were also documented for VRE infections in non-ICU patients. As of June 2004, 28.5% of ICU enterococcal isolates reported to the NNIS system were resistant to vancomycin.[17]

The North American Vancomycin Resistant Enterococci Susceptibility Study of 2002 (NAVRESS) demonstrated that VRE urinary isolates are disseminated throughout most regions of the United States and represent about 9.2% of all isolated enterococci.[18]

In the United States, the hospital is the primary reservoir for VRE, while in Europe VRE have been isolated from sewage and animal sources.[19,20] In 1994, a study by Bates and coworkers found a connection between the use of avoparcin—an animal growth promoter used in Europe

Table 4-2: Risk Factors for Colonization or Infection With VRE

- Prolonged hospitalization
- Serious illness
- Enteral tube feedings
- Prolonged ICU stay
- Exposure to contaminated medical equipment
- Proximity to known VRE patient
- Transplant recipients and hematology/oncology patients
- Intra-abdominal surgery
- Exposure to personnel caring for VRE patients
- Previous treatment with antibiotics

From Cetinkaya[3], Rice[4], Patel[14], and Huycke[26]

but not in the United States—and the development of VRE colonization in pigs and chickens. Further studies resulted in a European Union ban on avoparcin in 1997.

Characteristics of enterococci

Enterococci have characteristics that enhance their survival and they can tolerate a wide range of growth conditions. They can thrive in temperatures of 10°C to 45°C and can live in bile salts and sodium azide solutions. VRE are also capable of prolonged survival on environmental surfaces, patient-care equipment, hands, and gloves.[21,22] Some strains are resistant to almost all available antimicrobials.[7,23]

Of the two species of enterococci that cause the most human infections, *E faecalis* was reported in 80% to 90% of enterococcal infections and *E faecium* accounted for 5% to 10%.[23,24] However, 2001 data from the Sentry Antimicrobial Resistance Surveillance Program showed that *E faecium* infections increased to account for 20% of clinical enterococcal infections in the United States.[25] The *E faecium* species is less pathogenic than *E faecalis*, but is more likely to be vancomycin resistant. In fact, 95% of VRE in the United States are *E faecium*.[4]

Risk factors for VRE

Table 4-2 lists various risk factors that predispose patients to VRE infection. Among the antibiotics implicated in the development of VRE are clindamycin (Cleocin®), cephalosporins, aztreonam, ciprofloxacin (Cipro®), aminoglycosides, metronidazole, and vancomycin.[3,4,26] Studies indicate that the use of anti-anaerobic agents, such as clindamycin, is associated with the development of VRE.[27] A switch from ticarcillin/clavulanate (Timentin®) to piperacillin/tazobactam (Zosyn®) for treatment of VRE in another study resulted in a reduction in nosocomial acquisition of VRE and patient colonization.[28] Patients in long-term-care facilities have been shown to be reservoirs of VRE,[29] which means colonized patients transferred from a long-term-care facility to a hospital may transmit VRE within the hospital.

Costs associated with VRE

A meta-analysis by Salgado et al documented increased costs from VRE infections.[30] The study showed that VRE caused prolonged hospital stays, longer ICU stays, and higher mortality among VRE patients. Because VRE are typically resistant to β-lactam antibiotics, newer agents are generally needed for treatment, and these drugs are more costly than vancomycin.

Prevention and control

Studies have shown that VRE are transferred by patient-to-patient contact, via the hands of health-care workers, or from contaminated patient-care equipment or environmental sites.[31,32] The routine use of gowns and gloves instead of gloves alone showed significant benefits in a study on nosocomial transfer of VRE in an ICU.[33]

Table 4-3: Risk Index Score for Recovery of Vancomycin-Resistant Enterococci at Hospital Admission, by Associated Risk Factor

Risk Factor	Point Value
Previous recovery of MRSA*	4
Long-term hemodialysis	3
Transfer from LTCF or hospital	3
Exposure to ≥2 antibiotics**	3
Previous hospitalization*	3
Age >60 years	2

LTCF = long-term-care facility;
MRSA = methicillin-resistant *S aureus*
* Within 1 year of study enrollment
** Within 30 days of study enrollment
From Tacconelli[36]

In 1995, the Hospital Infection Control Practices Advisory Committee (HIPAC) formulated guidelines for managing VRE infections, titled Recommendations for Preventing the Spread of Vancomycin Resistance.[31] Key points of these guidelines include prudent vancomycin use, education programs for hospital staff, laboratory identification of enterococci at the species level (under special circumstances), and the development of protocols for screening for VRE. Periodic antimicrobial susceptibility testing is recommended for early detection of VRE and periodic culture surveys of stools or rectal swabs are recommended in hospitals that have many critically ill patients. Isolation precautions should be followed in hospitals where VRE is endemic.

In 2003, in addition to the HIPAC guidelines, the Society for Healthcare Epidemiology of America (SHEA) recommended active surveillance cultures as essential for identification of VRE reservoirs.[34] An interinstitutional study compared data from one hospital that practiced routine, active surveillance for VRE colonization in high-risk patients to data from another hospital that did not perform routine surveillance.[35] Routine surveillance showed a significantly lower rate of VRE bacteremia (more than twofold).

Tacconelli et al developed a clinical prediction rule to identify patients at high risk for having VRE colonization at hospital admission (Table 4-3).[36] Six variables were identified at admission and weighted scores were applied. When a cut-off value of ≥10 was used for the point score, the specificity of the prediction rule was 98% for risk of VRE colonization.

Clinical Infections

Although enterococci are of relatively low virulence, they are able to thrive in many environments that would kill most bacteria. Enterococci primarily cause urinary tract infections, bacteremia, endocarditis, wound infections, and intra-abdominal abscesses.[6,14,37,38]

Bacteremia is a life-threatening illness. Data from the SENTRY Antimicrobial Resistance Surveillance Program indicate that bacteremia is the third most frequent infection caused by enterococci.[22] Enterococci are also the third most prevalent pathogens causing nosocomial bloodstream infections in the United States.[22,39]

Risk factors for enterococcal bacteremia include prior antimicrobial administration, hemodialysis, surgery, indwelling urinary or vascular catheters, and treatment with corticosteroids, antineoplastic agents, or total parenteral nutrition.[40,41] Data collected by The Surveillance Network (TSN) in 2002 indicated six organisms, including both *E faecium* and *E faecalis*, accounted for >80% of all blood culture isolates[42] (Table 4-4).

Table 4-4: Frequencies of Occurrence of Bacterial Species or Groups Isolated From Blood Cultures of Hospitalized Patients in the US in 2002

Rank	Bacterial species or group
1	Coagulase-negative staphylococci
2	*S aureus*
3	*E faecalis*
4	*E coli*
5	*K pneumoniae*
6	*E faecium*

Adapted from Karlowsky[42]

The Surveillance and Control of Pathogens of Epidemiological Importance (SCOPE) study found that although only 9% of nosocomial bloodstream infections were caused by enterococci, vancomycin resistance was found in 60% of *E faecium* isolates (and 2% of *E faecalis* isolates), making antimicrobial treatment challenging.[43] Data for pediatric patients indicated 11% VRE for *E faecium* and 1% for *E faecalis*.[44]

Bloodstream infections can lead to bacterial endocarditis, especially in patients with pre-existing valvular abnormalities.[37] Surface adhesins on the circulating bacteria facilitate adherence to host epithelium, proteins, or thrombi, and platelet-fibrin vegetation is formed on valves. Organisms become caught in the vegetation and contribute to its growth. Once the bacteria are enclosed in the vegetation, host antibodies can no longer reach the bacteria.[45] Enterococci account for 10% to 20% of cases of

No. of isolates	% of total no. of isolates
34,640	42.0
13,618	16.5
6,893	8.3
5,942	7.2
0,942	3.6
2,873	3.5

bacteremic endocarditis on both native and prosthetic valves.[6] Enterococcal endocarditis is usually subacute but may be acute and damage the valves.

Liver abscesses may result as a complication of biliary surgery and other intra-abdominal infections may develop after surgery.[46] Intra-abdominal VRE infections have been associated with pancreatic pseudocysts, fecal peritonitis, and biliary sepsis after surgery for common bile duct stones.[46] VRE have been reported to cause peritonitis in continuous ambulatory peritoneal dialysis patients.[47] Pelvic infections and postpartum endomyometritis may also occur with enterococcal infections.

Enterococci rarely cause respiratory tract infections.[48] When enterococci are cultured from the respiratory tract, they generally represent colonization rather than infection.

Surgical wounds—especially if associated with intestinal surgery—decubitus ulcers, burns, and diabetic foot

Table 4-5: Antibiotic Activity Against VRE From Urinary Isolates

Antibiotic	% Susceptible	
	E faecium (VRE)	*E faecalis* (VRE)
ampicillin	3.2	97.5
chloramphenicol	99.1	77.8
doxycycline	60.7	35.8
vancomycin	0.0	0.0
gentamicin	56.8	18.5
streptomycin	28.9	44.4
linezolid	99.5	100.0
quinupristin/ dalfopristin	75.8	2.5
nitrofurantoin	95.8	98.8
ciprofloxacin	0.0	1.2
teicoplanin*	22.2	43.2

Adapted from Zhanel[18]
*Not approved in US.

ulcers may become infected with enterococci. Either endogenous intestinal flora or organisms from a fecally contaminated environment can be responsible for infecting tissue if epithelium is disrupted.[49]

Urinary tract infections (UTIs) are the most frequent infections caused by enterococci.[25] Most UTIs are nosocomial and associated with instrumentation of the genitourinary tract. Prior administration of antimicrobials is also a contributing factor to the development of enterococcal UTIs.[6] VRE can cause cystitis, pyelonephritis, perinephric abscess, and prostatitis.[14] Table 4-5 shows activity of various antimicrobials against VRE urinary isolates.

Treatment

Treatment of enterococcal infections begins with drainage of abscesses and debridement of wounds. Foreign bodies, such as intravascular catheters and indwelling urinary catheters, should be removed if they are sites of infection. In some cases, catheter removal alone is sufficient for resolution of line-related bacteremia.[50] However, there may be instances when the indwelling catheter cannot be removed, and in these cases patients require systemic antibiotic therapy.

Urinary tract infections caused by VRE can be treated with nitrofurantoin (Macrobid®, Macrodantin®, Furadantin®) or fosfomycin (Monurol®), if the isolates are susceptible.[38] These agents are effective for UTIs because they achieve adequate therapeutic levels in the urine. They do not, however, reach therapeutic levels in the blood and are, therefore, not useful for bacteremias or systemic infections. Fluoroquinolones have also shown effectiveness for uncomplicated UTIs from VRE that are caused by susceptible isolates.[38]

Antimicrobials for treatment of VRE bacteremia and systemic VRE infections are limited, but several antimicrobials have shown good activity against this organism. Quinupristin/dalfopristin and linezolid are approved drugs with indications for VRE, and daptomycin shows promise.

Quinupristin/dalfopristin

Quinupristin/dalfopristin (Synercid®) is a novel, intravenously administered antimicrobial that is a combination of two semisynthetic streptogramins with a 30:70 quinupristin:dalfopristin ratio. This synergistic combination inhibits protein synthesis of the bacterial ribosome. Resistance to quinupristin/dalfopristin is uncommon.[51]

One of quinupristin/dalfopristin's approved indications is for the treatment of patients with serious or life-threatening infections associated with vancomycin-resistant *E faecium* bacteremia (Table 4-6).[51] Quinupristin/dalfopristin is not, however, effective against *E faecalis*.

Table 4-6: Bacteriologic Response Rate to Treatment of VRE (*E faecium*) Infection With Intravenous Quinupristin/Dalfopristin

	Number of patients		
Indication	Enrolled (%)	Evaluable*	Response %
Intra-abdominal infection	135 (33.9)	56	58.9 (33/56)
Bacteremia of unknown origin	113 (28.9)	27	51.9 (14/27)
Urinary tract infection	35 (8.7)	18	88.9 (16/18)
Catheter-related bacteremia	32 (8.0)	12	83.3 (10/12)
Skin/skin structure infection	31 (8.0)	18	72.2 (13/18)
Bone and joint infection	13 (3.2)	6	83.3 (5/6)

*Bacteriologically evaluable
From Moellering[55]

Safety and tolerability data from clinical trials show that quinupristin/dalfopristin is metabolized by the cytochrome P-450 3A4 system.[52] The concomitant administration of quinupristin/dalfopristin and other drugs metabolized by cytochrome P-450 may result in higher plasma concentrations of these latter drugs, resulting in increased or prolonged therapeutic effect and/or increased adverse effects (Table 4-7). Although electrocardiograph studies show that quinupristin/dalfopristin itself does not cause prolongation

Table 4-7: Drugs That Can Have Increased Plasma Concentrations Following Concomitant Administration With Quinupristin/Dalfopristin*

• Antihistamines	astemizole
• Anti-HIV drugs	delavirdine, nevirapine, indinavir, ritonavir
• Antineoplastic agents	vinca alkaloids (eg, vinblastine), docetaxel, paclitaxel
• Benzodiazepines	midazolam, diazepam
• Calcium channel blockers	dihydropyridines (eg, nifedipine), verapamil, diltiazem
• Cholesterol-lowering agents	HMG-CoA reductase inhibitors (statins, eg, lovastatin)
• GI motility agents	cisapride
• Immunosuppressive agents	cyclosporine, tacrolimus
• Steroids	methylprednisolone
• Others	carbamazepine, quinidine, lidocaine, disopyramide

*This list of drugs is not all-inclusive
From Rubinstein[52]

of the QTc interval, administration of concomitant medications metabolized by cytochrome P-450 that may cause prolongation of QTc should be avoided.[52]

In a study by Raad et al,[53] myalgias/arthralgias in patients treated with quinupristin/dalfopristin were associated with biliary dysfunction. Reducing the dose of quinupristin/dalfopristin should be considered for patients with biliary dysfunction or those taking medications that can cause hepatic cholestasis.[54] Myalgias/arthralgias resolved when the drug was discontinued.

The recommended dosage of quinupristin/dalfopristin in adults is 7.5 mg/kg of body weight, administered by IV route in 5% glucose/dextrose solution over 60 minutes every 8 or 12 hours, depending on the site of infection.[52] Venous irritation is common when the antibiotic is administered via peripheral vein; therefore, a central venous catheter or a peripherally inserted central catheter is the preferred method of delivery. The most frequently reported treatment-related adverse effects with quinupristin/dalfopristin are arthralgia, myalgia, nausea, and pain.[55]

In vitro studies of quinupristin/dalfopristin with other antimicrobials, such as doxycycline or gentamicin, indicate enhanced activity, although clinical data are lacking.[56] A drawback to quinupristin/dalfopristin is that it is bacteriostatic against enterococci.[49]

Linezolid

In 2000, linezolid (Zyvox®) became the first licensed member of a new class of antibiotics, the oxazolidinones, which inhibit protein synthesis by blocking initiation complex formation. Because of this novel mechanism of action, oxazolidinones do not exhibit cross-resistance with other existing antibacterial agents.[57] Linezolid is rapidly absorbed with peak plasma concentration (C_{max}) achieved in 0.3 to 1 hour. Because it is not metabolized by the cytochrome P-450 3A4 enzyme system, linezolid is unlikely to interact with other drugs through induction or inhibition of that system.

Unlike quinupristin/dalfopristin, linezolid is active against both *E faecalis* and *E faecium*. Linezolid is available for either oral or IV administration and is 100%

bioavailable orally.[58] Oral administration has a distinct advantage for patients with severe infections and prolonged hospital stays, because the long-term vascular access needed for IV administration places a patient at increased risk for catheter-related infection.[59] Resistance to linezolid is uncommon and has only been reported in enterococcal infections.[58] Prolonged use of linezolid, however has been associated with the development of decreased vancomycin-resistant *E faecium* susceptibility.[53]

A number of in vitro studies have assessed linezolid activity. Jones et al[60] reported the in vitro susceptibility to linezolid of the major multidrug-resistant pathogens, including VRE. VRE was shown to be susceptible to linezolid at $MIC_{90} \leq 2$ μg/mL. Noskin et al tested linezolid against gram-positive bacteria, including *E faecium* and *E faecalis*.[58] All isolates were inhibited by linezolid at MIC ≤4 μg/mL, including VRE isolates. Additional studies resulted in linezolid inhibition of all isolates at concentrations between 1 and 4 μg/mL, regardless of resistance profile.[61,62] Using the approved dose of 600 mg every 12 hours results in serum linezolid concentrations of 6.15 to 21.12 μg/mL.

In a phase I study, Stalker et al[63] assessed the tolerability and pharmacokinetics of oral linezolid. The most frequently reported adverse effects were tongue discoloration, rash, and dermatitis. For IV linezolid, another phase I study by Stalker et al[64] found GI discomfort, tongue discoloration, and rash as the most commonly reported adverse effects.

A phase III study using a twice-daily dose of 600 mg showed cure rates of 79%, which were similar to the cure rates observed in subjects who were part of a linezolid compassionate use program.[65] Infection categories in the phase III study included urinary tract infections, skin and soft structure infections, bacteremia, peritonitis, intra-abdominal infections, catheter-related infections, and pneumonia. At follow-up, the group taking 600 mg linezolid twice a day (vs 200 mg) showed an 88% success rate.

Table 4-8: Incidence of Adverse Events Reported in ≥2% of Patients Treated With Linezolid

Event	Incidence, %
Diarrhea	8.3
Headache	6.5
Nausea	6.2
Vomiting	3.7
Insomnia	2.5
Constipation	2.2
Rash	2.0
Dizziness	2.0

From Zyvox® [package insert]. Kalamazoo, Mich, Pharmacia & Upjohn, 2000

An additional phase III study by Birmingham et al showed linezolid as effective for the treatment of bacteremia caused by gram-positive organisms.[66] Other studies indicate clinical efficacy in neutropenic patients[67] and for outpatients with resistant gram-positive infections.[68]

Burn victims are at high risk for developing VRE and infections with multidrug-resistant organisms because of prolonged hospital stay, exposure to broad-spectrum antibiotic therapy, and immunocompromised status from the burns.[69] Treatment involves both antibiotic therapy and surgical intervention to prevent serious complications, such as delayed wound healing and skin graft breakdown, which may lead to loss of an affected limb or even death.

In a study by Broder et al[69] of 40 patients who received linezolid for infections of wound coverage, the clinical success rate of linezolid with adjunct wound-coverage techniques was 100% for skin and soft tissue infections, 90.0% for osteomyelitis, and 83.3% for wound-coverage infections, such as graft or flap. Linezolid was well tolerated in 80% of the patients, with GI disturbances (nausea, vomiting, diarrhea) and dermatological reactions the most frequently reported adverse events. Table 4-8 lists the incidence of the most common adverse events for linezolid.

Bacteremic infections are serious complications in solid organ transplant recipients. The incidence of VRE infections and colonization range from 10.5%[70] to 18%[71] of all transplants, and VRE infections are associated with high mortality rates of up to 83%.[70,71] El Khoury and Fishman[72] evaluated 85 patients with solid organ transplants and documented VRE infections for response to linezolid treatment in an open-label, 53-center study. In linezolid-treated patients, mortality rates associated with VRE infection were 32.9% in the overall patient population, and in liver transplant recipients the rate was 42%.[70,71] Previous reports indicated a mortality rate of 53% to 83% in liver transplant patients who had not received linezolid.[70,71] Because linezolid is not cleared by either the kidneys or liver, dosage adjustment is not necessary in patients with kidney or liver dysfunction.[72]

Infective endocarditis is a rare complication of solid organ transplants, although the incidence is increasing.[59] In recent studies, gram-positive organisms, including two known cases of VRE, were the most frequently isolated organisms in infective endocarditis.

In addition to thrombocytopenia associated with linezolid treatment,[73,74] a few cases of serotonin syndrome have been reported, indicating linezolid may potentially interact with selective serotonin uptake inhibitors.[75] As a weak monoamine oxidase inhibitor, linezolid can potentiate adrenergic effects of pseudoephedrine or phenylpropanolamine, with the result of a mean increase in systolic blood pressure. Patients receiving linezolid should be advised, therefore, to avoid adrenergic agents, including foods or beverages with high tyramine content. In some patients, persistent optic and peripheral neuropathy have also been reported.[76]

Daptomycin

Daptomycin (Cubicin®) is the first member of another new class of antimicrobial drugs, the cyclic lipopeptides. In 2003, the US Food and Drug Administration (FDA) approved daptomycin for the treatment of complicated skin and skin-structure infections.[77] Daptomycin has potent bactericidal activity against a broad range of gram-positive pathogens and a low potential for resistance. Although the approved indications include only vancomycin-susceptible strains of *E faecalis*, studies show daptomycin to be bactericidal against VRE at concentrations near the MIC.[78,79] In vitro studies have also shown synergistic action of daptomycin with aminoglycosides or rifampicin.[80] Further studies are underway, which may provide dosing regimen suggestions for additional indications for daptomycin against drug-resistant gram-positive bacteria.[81]

Daptomycin's concentration-dependent activity allows for a once-daily regimen and reduces the probability of accumulation-related effects.[82] Daptomycin is administered at 4 mg/kg over a 30-minute period by IV infusion in 0.9% sodium chloride.[83] The most common adverse events for daptomycin from phase III trials include constipation, nausea, injection site reactions, headache, diarrhea, insomnia, and rash.[78] Additionally, elevations in serum creatine phosphokinase (CPK) were reported in phase III trials and skeletal muscle effects were observed in animal studies.[83] Because of the risk of myelopathy, it is recommended that patients receiving daptomycin be monitored for development of muscle pain or weakness. Also, CPK levels should be monitored weekly.

Investigational antimicrobials

Two investigational glycopeptides, dalbavancin and oritavancin, are being evaluated in phase II and III trials.[84,85] Both drugs have long half-lives, which has the advantage of less frequent dosing, rapid bactericidal activity, and diminished likelihood for development of resistance. Dalbavancin is a derivative of teicoplanin, which is a glycopeptide that is used in Europe but is not available in the United States. Oritavancin is a derivative of vancomycin.[86] The spectrum of activity for oritavancin includes VRE strains. Clinical studies are evaluating efficacy and safety for dalbavancin and oritavancin for the treatment of SSSIs and bacteremia, with once-daily administration for oritavancin and once weekly dosing for dalbavancin.[86]

Ramoplanin is the first glycolipodepsipeptide in clinical trials.[38,84] It interferes with bacterial cell-wall synthesis and is bactericidal against gram-positive bacteria only, including all strains of *E faecium* and *E faecalis*.[38] Ramoplanin is a promising agent for GI tract decolonization of VRE. It is being evaluated in phase III trials for the prevention of bacteremia in VRE-colonized patients.[14,84]

Tigecycline (Tygacil™) is a minocycline derivative that is a member of a new class of antimicrobials, the glycylcyclines. In vitro, tigecycline has exhibited excellent activity against gram-positive cocci, including VRE.[87] This antibiotic has received FDA approval for complicated skin, skin structure infections, and complicated intra-abdominal infections. Tigecycline is currently being evaluated for safety and efficacy in community-acquired pneumonia and hospital-acquired pneumonia.

References

1. Jett BD, Huycke MM, Gilmore MS: Virulence of enterococci. *Clin Microbiol Rev* 1994;7:462-478.

2. Mundy LM, Sahm DF, Gilmore M: Relationships between enterococcal virulence and antimicrobial resistance. *Clin Microbiol Rev* 2000;13:513-522.

3. Cetinkaya Y, Falk P, Mayhall CG: Vancomycin-resistant enterococci. *Clin Microbiol Rev* 2000;13:686-707.

4. Rice LB: Emergence of vancomycin-resistant enterococci. *Emerg Infect Dis* 2001;7:183-187.

5.   Frieden TR, Munsiff SS, Low DE, et al: Emergence of van-comycin-resistant enterococci in New York City. *Lancet* 1993;342:76-79.

6.   Wessels MR: Streptococcal and enterococcal infections. In: Braunwald E, Fauci AS, Kasper DL, et al, eds. *Harrison's Principles of Internal Medicine*, 15th ed. New York, NY, McGraw-Hill, 2001, pp 901-909.

7.   DeLisle S, Perl TM: Vancomycin-resistant enterococci: a road map on how to prevent the emergence and transmission of antimicrobial resistance. *Chest* 2003;123 (5 suppl):504S-518S.

8.   Grayson ML, Thauvin-Eliopoulos C, Eliopoulos GM, et al: Failure of trimethoprim-sulfamethoxazole therapy in experimental enterococcal endocarditis. *Antimicrob Agents Chemother* 1990;34:1792-1794.

9.   Murray BE: β-lactamase-producing enterococci. *Antimicrob Agents Chemother* 1992;36:2355-2359.

10.   Moellering RC Jr, Weinberg AN: Studies on antibiotic synergism against enterococci. II. Effect of various antibiotics on uptake of 14C-labeled streptomycin by enterococci. *J Clin Investig* 1971;50:2580-2584.

11.   Woodford N, Johnson AP, Morrison D, et al: Current perspectives on glycopeptide resistance. *Clin Microbiol Rev* 1995;8:584-615.

12.   Johnson AP: The pathogenicity of enterococci. *J Antimicrob Chemother* 1994;33:1083-1089.

13.   Isenmann R, Schwarz M, Rozdzinski E, et al: Interaction of fibronectin and aggregation substance promotes adherence of *Enterococcus faecalis* to human colon. *Dig Dis Sci* 2002;47:462-468.

14.   Patel R: Clinical impact of vancomycin-resistant enterococci. *J Antimicrob Chemother* 2003;(suppl 51):iii13-iii21.

15.   Sandoe JA, Witherden IR, Cove JH, et al: Correlation between enterococcal biofilm formation in vitro and medical-device-related infection potential in vivo. *J Med Microbiol* 2003;52:547-550.

16.   Centers for Disease Control and Prevention: Nosocomial enterococci resistant to vancomycin-United States, 1989-1993. *MMWR Morb Mortal Wkly Rep* 1993;42:597-599.

17.   National Nosocomial Infections Surveillance (NNIS) System Report: Data summary from January 1992 through June 2004, issued October 2004. *Am J Infect Control* 2004;32:470-485.

18. Zhanel GG, Laing NM, Nichol KA, et al: Antibiotic activity against urinary tract infection (UTI) isolates of vancomycin-resistant enterococci (VRE): results from the 2002 North American Vancomycin Resistant Enterococci Susceptibility Study. (NAVRESS). *J Antimicrob Chemother* 2003;52:382-388.

19. Bates J, Jordens JZ, Griffiths DT: Farm animals as a putative reservoir for vancomycin-resistant enterococcal infection in man. *J Antimicrob Chemother* 1994;34:507-514.

20. Klare I, Heier H, Claus H, et al: *Enterococcus faecium* strains with vanA-mediated high-level glycopeptide resistance isolated from foodstuffs and fecal samples of humans in the community. *Microb Drug Resist* 1995;1:265-272.

21. Noskin GA, Stosor V, Cooper I, et al: Recovery of vancomycin-resistant enterococci on fingertips and environmental surfaces. *Infect Control Hosp Epidemiol* 1995;16:577-581.

22. Noskin GA, Bednarz P, Suriano T, et al: Persistent contamination of fabric-covered furniture by vancomycin-resistant enterococci: implications for upholstery selection in hospitals. *Am J Infect Control* 2000;28:311-313.

23. Gold HS: Vancomycin-resistant enterococci: mechanisms and clinical observations. *Clin Infect Dis* 2001;33:210-219.

24. Treitman AN, Yarnold PR, Warren J, et al: Emerging incidence of *Enterococcus faecium* among hospital isolates (1993 to 2002). *J Clin Microbiol* 2005;43:462-463.

25. Low DE, Keller N, Barth A, et al: Clinical prevalence, antimicrobial susceptibility, and geographic resistance patterns of enterococci: results from the SENTRY Antimicrobial Surveillance Program, 1997-1999. *Clin Infect Dis* 2001;32:S133-S145.

26. Huycke MM, Sahm DF, Gilmore MS: Multiple-drug resistant enterococci: the nature of the problem and an agenda for the future. *Emerg Infect Dis* 1998;4:239-249.

27. Lautenbach E, LaRosa LA, Marr AM, et al: Changes in the prevalence of vancomycin-resistant enterococci in response to antimicrobial formulary interventions: impact of progressive restrictions on use of vancomycin and third-generation cephalosporins. *Clin Infect Dis* 2003;36:440-446.

28. Winston LG, Charlebois ED, Pang S, et al: Impact of a formulary switch from ticarcillin-clavulanate to piperacillin-tazobactam on colonization with vancomycin-resistant enterococci. *Am J Infect Control* 2004;32:462-469.

29. Elizaga ML, Weinstein RA, Hayden MK: Patients in long-term care facilities: a reservoir for vancomycin-resistant enterococci. *Clin Infect Dis* 2002;34:441-446.

30. Salgado CD, Farr BM: Outcomes associated with vancomycin-resistant enterococci: a meta-analysis. *Infect Control Hosp Epidemiol* 2003;24:690-698.

31. Centers for Disease Control and Prevention: Recommendations for preventing the spread of vancomycin resistance. Recommendations of the Hospital Infection Control Practices Advisory Committee (HIPAC). *MMWR Morb Mortal Wkly Rep* 1995;44:RR-12.

32. Duckro AN, Blom DW, Lyle EA, et al: Transfer of vancomycin-resistant enterococci via health care worker hands. *Arch Intern Med* 2005;165:302-307.

33. Srinivasan A, Song X, Ross T, et al: A prospective study to determine whether cover gowns in addition to gloves decrease nosocomial transmission of vancomycin-resistant enterococci in an intensive care unit. *Infect Control Hosp Epidemiol* 2002;23:424-428.

34. Muto CA, Jernigan JA, Ostrowsky BE, et al: SHEA guideline for preventing nosocomial transmission of multidrug-resistant strains of *Staphylococcus aureus* and enterococcus. *Infect Control Hosp Epidemiol* 2003;24:362-386.

35. Price CS, Paule S, Noskin GA, et al: Active surveillance reduces the incidence of vancomycin-resistant enterococcal bacteremia. *Clin Infect Dis* 2003;37:921-928.

36. Tacconelli E, Karchmer AW, Yokoe D, et al: Preventing the influx of vancomycin-resistant enterococci into health care institutions, by use of a simple validated prediction rule. *Clin Infect Dis* 2004;39:964-970.

37. Chambers HF: Infectious diseases: bacterial and chlamydial. In: Tierney LM Jr, McPhee SJ, Papadakis MA, eds. *Current Medical Diagnosis and Treatment*, 43rd ed. New York, NY Lange Medical Books/McGraw-Hill, 2004, pp 1337-1379.

38. Kauffman CA: Therapeutic and preventative options for the management of vancomycin-resistant enterococcal infections. *J Antimicrob Chemother* 2003;51(suppl 3)iii23-iii30.

39. Karchmer AW: Nosocomial bloodstream infections: organisms, risk factors, and implications. *Clin Infect Dis* 2000;31:S139-S143.

40. Peset V, Tallon P, Sola C, et al: Epidemiological, microbiological, clinical, and prognostic factors of bacteremia caused by high-level vancomycin-resistant *Enterococcus* species. *Eur J Clin Microbiol Infect Dis* 2000;19:742-749.

41. Vergis EN, Hayden MK, Chow JW, et al: Determinants of vancomycin resistance and mortality rates in enterococcal bacteremia. A prospective multicenter study. *Ann Intern Med* 2001;135:484-492.

42. Karlowsky JA, Jones ME, Draghi DC, et al: Prevalence and antimicrobial susceptibilities of bacteria isolated from blood cultures of hospitalized patients in the United States in 2002. *Ann Clin Microbiol Antimicrob* 2004;3:7.

43. Wisplinghoff H, Bischoff T, Tallent SM, et al: Nosocomial bloodstream infections in US hospitals: analysis of 24,179 cases from a prospective nationwide surveillance study. *Clin Infect Dis* 2004;39:309-317.

44. Wisplinghoff H, Seifert H, Tallent SM, ct al: Nosocomial bloodstream infections in pediatric patients in United States hospitals: epidemiology, clinical features and susceptibilities. *Pediatr Infect Dis J* 2003;22:686-691.

45. McCormick JK, Tripp TJ, Dunny GM, et al: Formation of vegetations during infective endocarditis excludes binding of bacterial-specific host antibodies to *Enterococcus faecalis*. *J Infect Dis* 2002;185:994-997.

46. Poduval RD, Kamath RP, Corpuz M, et al: Intra-abdominal vancomycin-resistant *Enterococcus* infections: the new threat. *J Clin Gastroenterol* 2001;32:333-335.

47. Zaleznik DR, Kasper DL: Intra-abdominal infections and abscesses. In: Braunwald E, Fauci AS, Kasper DL, et al, eds. *Harrison's Principles of Internal Medicine*, 15th ed. New York, NY, McGraw-Hill, 2001, pp 829-834.

48. Murray BE: Diversity among multidrug-resistant enterococci. *Emerg Infect Dis* 1998;4:37-47.

49. Levison ME, Mallela S: Increasing antimicrobial resistance: therapeutic implications for enterococcal infections. *Curr Infect Dis Rep* 2000;2:417-423.

50. Lai KK: Treatment of vancomycin-resistant *Enterococcus faecium* infections. *Arch Intern Med* 1996;156:2579-2584.

51. Eliopoulos GM: Quinupristin-dalfopristin and linezolid: evidence and opinion. *Clin Infect Dis* 2003;36:473-481.

52. Rubinstein E, Prokocimer P, Talbot GH: Safety and tolerability of quinupristin/dalfopristin: administration guidelines. *J Antimicrob Chemother* 1999;44:37-46.

53. Raad II, Hanna HA, Hachem RY, et al: Clinical-use-associated decrease in susceptibility of vancomycin-resistant *Enterococcus faecium* to linezolid: a comparison with quinupristin-dalfopristin. *Antimicrob Agents Chemother* 2004;48:3583-3585.

54. Raad I, Hachem R, Hanna H, et al: Prospective, randomized study comparing quinupristin-dalfopristin with linezolid in the treatment of vancomycin-resistant *Enterococcus faecium* infections. *J Antimicrob Chemother* 2004;53:646-649.

55. Moellering RC: Quinupristin/dalfopristin: therapeutic potential for vancomycin-resistant enterococcal infections. *J Antimicrob Chemother* 1999;44:25-30.

56. Eliopoulos GM, Wennersten CB: Antimicrobial activity of quinupristin-dalfopristin combined with other antibiotics against vancomycin-resistant enterococci. *Antimicrob Agents Chemother* 2002;46:1319-1324.

57. Hamel JC, Stapert D, Moerman JK, et al: Linezolid, critical characteristics. *Infection* 2000;28:60-64.

58. Noskin GA, Siddiqui F, Stosor V, et al: In vitro activities of linezolid against important gram-positive bacterial pathogens including vancomycin-resistant enterococci. *Antimicrob Agents Chemother* 1999;43:2059-2062.

59. Archuleta S, Murphy B, Keller MJ: Successful treatment of vancomycin-resistant *Enterococcus faecium* endocarditis with linezolid in a renal transplant recipient with human immunodeficiency virus infection. *Transpl Infect Dis* 2004;6:117-119.

60. Jones RN, Pfaller MA, Erwin ME, et al: Antimicrobial activity of linezolid tested against 3808 strains of gram-positive organisms having resistances to various drugs. In: Program and abstracts of the 37th Annual Meeting of the Infectious Diseases Society of America; November 18-21, 1999, Philadelphia, PA.

61. Eliopoulos GM, Wennersten CB, Gold HS, et al: In vitro activities of new oxazolidinone antimicrobial agents against enterococci. *Antimicrob Agents Chemother* 1996;40:1745-1747.

62. Mezzatesta ML, Stefani S, Tempera G, et al: Comparative activity of linezolid against staphylococci and enterococci isolated in Italy. In: Program and Abstracts of the 40th Interscience Conference on Antimicrobial Agents and Chemotherapy, September 17-20, 2000, Toronto, Ontario, Canada. Abstract 2302.

63. Stalker DJ, Wajszczuk CP, Batts DH: Linezolid safety, tolerance and pharmacokinetics following oral dosing twice daily for 14.5 days. In: Program and abstracts of the 37th Interscience Conference on Antimicrobial Agents and Chemotherapy, September 28-October 1, 1997, Toronto, Ontario, Canada. Abstract A-115.

64. Stalker DJ, Wajszczuk CP, Batts DH: Linezolid safety, tolerance and pharmacokinetics after intravenous dosing twice daily for 7.5 days. In: Program and abstracts of the 37th Interscience Conference on Antimicrobial Agents and Chemotherapy; September 28-October 1, 1997; Toronto, Ontario, Canada. Abstract A-116.

65. Birmingham MC, Zimmer GS, Hafkin B, et al: Outcomes with linezolid from an ongoing compassionate use trial of patients with significant, resistant, gram-positive infections. In: Abstracts of the 39th Inter-Science Conference on Antimicrobial Agents and Chemotherapy, San Francisco, CA, 1999. Abstract 1098, p 724. American Society for Microbiology, Washington, DC.

66. Birmingham MC, Zimmer GS, Hafkin B, et al: Results of treating bacteremic patients with linezolid in a compassionate use trial for resistant gram-positive infections. In: Program and Abstracts of the 37th Annual Meeting of the Infectious Diseases Society of America, November 18-21, 1999, Philadelphia, PA.

67. Smith PF, Birmingham MC, Zimmer GS, et al: Clinical outcomes, safety and tolerance of linezolid for resistant gram-positive infections in patients with neutropenia. In: Program and Abstracts of the 37th Annual Meeting of the Infectious Diseases Society of America, November 18-21, 1999, Philadelphia, PA.

68. Birmingham MC, Rayner CR, Flavin SM, et al: Treating outpatients with significant resistant gram-positive infections with linezolid. In: Program and Abstracts of the 38th Annual Meeting of the Infectious Diseases Society of America, September 7-10, 2000, New Orleans, LA. Abstract 61.

69. Broder KW, Moise PA, Schultz RO, et al: Clinical experience with linezolid in conjunction with wound coverage techniques for skin and soft-tissue infections and postoperative osteomyelitis. *Ann Plast Surg* 2004;52:385-390.

70. Newell KA, Millis JM, Arnow PM, et al: Incidence and outcome of infection by vancomycin-resistant *Enterococcus* following orthotopic liver transplantation. *Transplantation* 1998;65:439-442.

71. Orloff SL, Busch AM, Olyaei AJ, et al: Vancomycin-resistant *Enterococcus* in liver transplant patients. *Am J Surg* 1999;177:418-422.

72. El-Khoury J, Fishman JA: Linezolid in the treatment of vancomycin-resistant *Enterococcus faecium* in solid organ transplant recipients: report of a multicenter compassionate-use trial. *Transpl Infect Dis* 2003;5:121-125.

73. Rao N, Ziran BH, Wagener MM, et al: Similar hematologic effects of long-term linezolid and vancomycin therapy in a prospective observational study of patients with orthopedic devices. *Clin Infect Dis* 2004;38:1058-1064.

74. Legout L, Senneville E, Gomel JJ, et al: Linezolid-induced neuropathy. *Clin Infect Dis* 2004;38:767-768.

75. Wigen CL, Goetz MB: Serotonin syndrome and linezolid. *Clin Infect Dis* 2002;34:1651-1652.

76. Frippiat F, Bergiers C, Michel C, et al: Severe bilateral optic neuritis associated with prolonged linezolid therapy. *J Antimicrob Agents Chemother* 2004;32:137-143.

77. Eisenstein BI: Lipopeptides, focusing on daptomycin, for the treatment of gram-positive infections. *Expert Opin Investig Drugs* 2004;13:1159-1169.

78. Steenbergen JN, Alder J, Thorne GM, et al: Daptomycin: a lipopeptide antibiotic for the treatment of serious gram-positive infections. *J Antimicrob Chemother* 2005;55:283-288.

79. Streit JM, Fritsche TR, Sader HS, et al: Worldwide assessment of dalbavancin activity and spectrum against over 6,000 clinical isolates. *Diagn Microbiol Infect Dis* 2004;48:137-143.

80. Rand KH, Houck H: Daptomycin synergy with rifampicin and ampicillin against vancomycin-resistant enterococci. *J Antimicrob Chemother* 2004;53:530-532.

81. Safdar N, Andes D, Craig WA: In vivo pharmacodynamic activity of daptomycin. *Antimicrob Agents Chemother* 2004;48:63-68.

82. Tally FP, DeBruin MF: Development of daptomycin for gram-positive infections. *J Antimicrob Chemother* 2000;46:523-526.

83. Cubicin® [package insert]. Lexington, MA: Cubist Pharmaceuticals, 2003.

84. Torres-Viera C, Dembry LM: Approaches to vancomycin-resistant enterococci. *Curr Opin Infect Dis* 2004;17:541-547.

85. Raghavan M, Linden PK: Newer treatment options for skin and soft tissue infections. *Drugs* 2004;64:1621-1642.

86. Van Bambeke F: Glycopeptides in clinical development: pharmacological profile and clinical perspectives. *Curr Opin Pharmacol* 2004;4:471-478.

87. Milatovic D, Schmitz FJ, Verhoef J, et al: Activities of the glycylcycline tigecycline (GAR-936) against 1,924 recent European clinical bacterial isolates. *Antimicrob Agents Chemother* 2003;47:400-404.

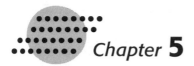 Chapter **5**

Acinetobacter

*A*cinetobacter species are generally not considered virulent pathogens, but because they have developed resistance to multiple antibiotics, they have become formidable foes worldwide. *Acinetobacter* organisms are mainly nosocomial pathogens, causing a wide range of clinical infections, including pneumonia, bacteremia, endocarditis, peritonitis, meningitis, soft-tissue infections, and urinary tract infections.[1] Carbapenems such as imipenem and meropenem (Merrem®) have been the treatments of choice, especially for multidrug-resistant *Acinetobacter* species. But carbapenem-resistant *Acinetobacter* species have been reported from France, Spain, Argentina, Brazil, England, Hong Kong, Kuwait, Singapore, and Belgium, as well as the United States. The emergence of carbapenem resistance has triggered the search for other options for treatment of *Acinetobacter* species, including reevaluation of older agents and use of antibiotic combinations.

Clinical Microbiology

Acinetobacter organisms are gram-negative, nonfermentative, nonmotile, aerobic bacteria. They are catalase positive and oxidase negative. Because they are rod-shaped during the growth phase but cocci-shaped in the stationary phase, they are described as coccobacilli. The organisms are free-living and are found on animate and inanimate objects. They are widely dispersed in nature and are typically found in soil and water samples. An important survival feature is their ability to use a variety of carbon sources for growth.

The name 'Acinetobacter' has evolved through numerous taxonomic identities since the first species was likely first described in 1908 as *Diplococcus mucosus*.[2] Subsequent nomenclature focused on characteristics of the bacterium for description: achromacolor (colorless), anitratus (nitrate-nonreducing), and mima (mimics). Other names formerly applied to *Acinetobacter* species were *Bacterium anitratum, Herellea vaginicola, Mima polymorpha, Alcaligenes, Micrococcus calcoaceticus, Moraxella glucidolytica*, and *Moraxella lwoffii*. Identifying and standardizing species has been an ongoing process since the 1980s, when just one species, *Acinetobacter calcoaceticus*, was named with two subspecies, *anitratus* and *lwoffii*. At present, at least 19 different *Acinetobacter* strains or genomic species have been identified. Of these, *Acinetobacter baumannii* is a major nosocomial pathogen that is increasingly common among critically ill patients in intensive care units (ICUs).

The Gram-negative Cell

The cellular structure of gram-negative bacteria differs from that of gram-positive bacteria. Gram-negative cells have a thinner peptidoglycan layer that is linked to an outer membrane by a lipoprotein.[3] Proteins embedded in the outer membrane serve a variety of important functions. They regulate diffusion of molecules into the cell and maintain the integrity of the outer membrane. They also act as receptors for bacteriophages and assist in the transport of iron into the cell.

The outer membrane contains a lipopolysaccharide (LPS) layer, which is a major virulence factor. The lipid portion of the LPS contains lipid A, an endotoxin that is responsible for most of the harmful effects of the bacterium.[3] The outer membrane also contains porins, which are proteins that create water-filled channels for transport of hydrophilic molecules. The periplasmic space separates the outer membrane from the peptidoglycan layer and

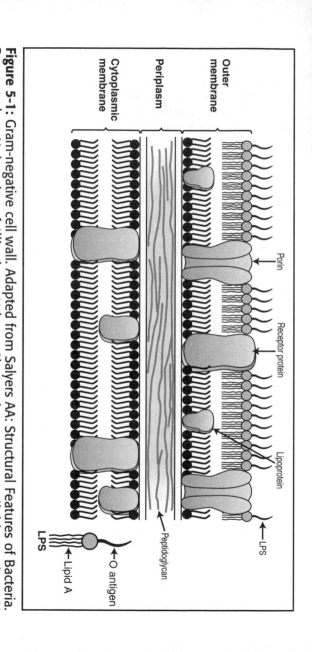

Figure 5-1: Gram-negative cell wall. Adapted from Salyers AA: Structural Features of Bacteria. Presented at University of Illinois at Urbana-Champaign, 2005. Available at: http://www.life.uiuc.edu/mcb/300/lectures/topic_04.ppt.

stores degradative enzymes (Figure 5-1). Most *Acineto-bacter* species also have a polysaccharide capsule, which is another protective mechanism. The capsule confers resistance to phagocytosis by blocking opsonization.

Mechanisms of Resistance

Acinetobacter species are resistant to desiccation, allowing the bacteria to survive for long periods on dry surfaces. This feature may explain why *Acinetobacter* sometimes causes extended outbreaks in the health-care setting. *Acinetobacter* species also tend to rapidly develop resistance to antimicrobials.[4] Mechanisms of antimicrobial resistance include low permeability of the outer membrane, altered penicillin-binding proteins, target site mutations, and inactivation of modifying enzymes.[4]

The major mechanism of resistance to β-lactam antibiotics is the production of β-lactamase. Several different enzymes are responsible for hydrolyzing β-lactam antibiotics, including carbapenems.[4]

Quinolone resistance is achieved by alteration of the target sites via chromosomal mutations. Enzymatic alteration is the mechanism of resistance against aminoglycosides. Reduction of uptake is another common mode of resistance in *Acinetobacter* species.

Pathogenesis and Virulence

Acinetobacter organisms are opportunistic. Unless normal host defense mechanisms are impaired, *Acinetobacter* species are generally not virulent. Host complement and phagocytosis are important defenses against invasion of pathogens. However, pathogenic bacteria can stimulate complement to the point that it becomes a liability to the host, resulting in tissue damage and shock.[5]

Pathogenesis

Patients susceptible to *Acinetobacter* infection include those with severe underlying conditions such as malignancy, burns, or immunosuppression and those undergoing surgical procedures. Extended stay in an ICU, espe-

Table 5-1: Typical Risk Factors for *Acinetobacter* Isolation From Two Teaching Hospitals

Risk Factors	HRAB (n = 84)	Control (n = 20)*	P value
Prior antibiotic usage	60	9	.035
Cardiovascular	49	12	1
ICU stay	41	5	.079
Nursing home residency	29	4	.288
Surgery	37	8	.806
Prior hospitalization	20	3	.553
Diabetes	18	8	.094
Malignancy	12	2	1
Respiratory	12	4	.504
Steroids	8	3	.439
Neurology	8	6	.026
Trauma	6	0	.593
Mechanical ventilation	47	6	.047
Tracheotomy	37	6	.317

HRAB = highly resistant *Acinetobacter baumannii*
ICU = intensive care unit
* The control group consisted of patients with 20 sensitive strains of *A baumannii*.
Adapted from Mahgoub et al, *Am J Infect Control* 2002;30:386-390.

cially with use of mechanical ventilation, and previous antimicrobial therapy, also predisposes patients to *Acinetobacter* infections (Table 5-1).[4,6]

Once the pathogen enters the host, adhesins produced by the bacterium bind the microbe to the host epithelium. The presence of fimbriae in some strains enhances adherence.[7] Fimbriae appear to be present only during the early, growth phase of *Acinetobacter* and are shed in later, stationary phases.

Virulence Factors

Although *Acinetobacter* organisms are considered low-virulence pathogens, they possess factors that increase the virulence of infective strains. The capsular polysaccharide present in most strains of *Acinetobacter* inhibits phagocytosis by preventing host opsonins from coating the microbes, a process that is necessary for uptake by phagocytosis.

The outer membrane of gram-negative bacteria, including *Acinetobacter*, is embedded with proteins that carry out various protective functions. Some proteins maintain the integrity of the outer membrane by acting as a selective barrier to penetration, and others act as receptors for bacteriophages or bind siderophores that transport iron into the bacterial cell.[3]

Endotoxin lipid A is present in the LPS component of the outer cell membrane.[2,3] The lipid A portion of LPS stimulates the production of inflammatory cytokines. Additional functions of LPS include resistance to bacteriolytic effects of complement and protection against antimicrobial defensins. Defensins kill bacteria and are found in high concentrations in myeloid cells, including platelets.[3]

One strain of *Acinetobacter*, *A calcoaceticus*, produces lipolytic enzymes that may damage tissue lipids.[8]

Epidemiology

The prevalence of *Acinetobacter* species varies by country but has increased overall in the last 2 decades.[2] *Acinetobacter* organisms have emerged as important health care-associated pathogens worldwide (Table 5-2).[1] Several characteristics of *Acinetobacter* species make them difficult to treat: they are free-living, are able to use a variety of carbon sources for growth,[2] tend to rapidly de-

Table 5-2: Prevalence of *Acinetobacter* Species in North America Versus Latin America

United States and Canada	Latin America
Acinetobacter baumannii: 54.6%	*A baumannii:* 75%
Acinetobacter anitratus: 14.8%	*A anitratus:* 8.2%
Acinetobacter calcoaceticus: 14.6%	*Acinetobacter* species: 7.4%

From Gales et al, *Clin Infect Dis* 2001;32(suppl 2):S104-S113, and the SENTRY Antimicrobial Surveillance Program, 1997-1999.

velop resistance to multiple antimicrobials,[4] and can survive for long periods in the hospital environment, which may facilitate person-to-person transmission.[6,9] *A baumannii* has been reported to survive up to 25 days on dry surfaces.[4]

Although some cases of community-acquired infections caused by *Acinetobacter* have been reported,[10,11] most infections are nosocomially acquired by immunocompromised or debilitated patients. *Acinetobacter* infection is most common in ICUs among mechanically ventilated patients and in long-term care facilities.[9]

One study cited *Acinetobacter* organisms as the most common gram-negative organisms persistently carried on the skin of hospital personnel.[12] They are also prevalent in moist areas of the body, such as the axillae, groin, and between the toes.[6] High rates of colonization of the skin, throat, and respiratory and digestive tracts have been documented in several hospital outbreaks, and colonization of the respiratory tract in particular has been associated with mechanically ventilated patients in ICUs.[13]

Because *Acinetobacter* species are known to survive for long periods on dry surfaces, the hospital environment is a reservoir for these organisms. *Acinetobacter* organisms have been recovered from sink traps, floors, and bedside cupboards in the rooms occupied by colonized patients.[14] Pillows, mattresses, bed linen, and curtains have also tested positive for *Acinetobacter* after discharge of colonized patients.

Many different classes of antimicrobials were successfully used to treat *Acinetobacter* infections until the organisms developed resistance to multiple classes of antibiotics. The first hospital outbreaks of multiple-drug-resistant *Acinetobacter* were described about 10 years ago.[15] Carbapenems, and especially imipenem, became the drugs of choice for infections with these resistant isolates, but imipenem-resistant strains quickly followed. In recent years, carbapenem-resistant *Acinetobacter* has increased worldwide.[1]

SENTRY Antimicrobial Surveillance Program

The SENTRY Antimicrobial Surveillance Program is an international surveillance program that monitors the frequency of occurrence and the antimicrobial susceptibilities of pathogens in sentinel hospitals. With respect to *Acinetobacter* infections, *A baumannii* was the species most commonly reported in three geographic regions evaluated in a report by Gales et al. Comparing the occurrence by region of various sites of *Acinetobacter* infection, analysis indicated that for the United States and Canada, isolates were frequently recovered from wounds and respiratory sites, whereas in Latin America, respiratory tract isolates were twice as frequent as wound isolates (Table 5-3).

National Nosocomial Infections Surveillance System

Data from the National Nosocomial Infections Surveillance System (NNIS) from 1992 through 1997 showed that *Acinetobacter* species caused 1% of nosocomial bloodstream infections (BSIs) and 3% of pneumonia cases in coronary care units.[16] Analysis of NNIS data between

**Table 5-3: Percentage of *Acinetobacter*
Species Observed by
Site of Infection***

Country or region	Blood
Canada	
Total no. of isolates	3,840
Acinetobacter %	0.7
(range)	(0.5-1.0)
United States	
Total no. of isolates	17,399
Acinetobacter %	1.4
(range)	(0.9-1.7)
Latin America	
Total no. of isolates	5,295
Acinetobacter %	4.6
(range)	(3.2-5.3)

* As reported in the SENTRY antimicrobial surveillance program, January 1997-December 1999.
From Gales et al, *Clin Infect Dis* 2001;32(suppl 2):S104-S113.

1987 and 1996 indicated a persistent seasonal increase during late summer months, possibly related to increased humidity, which favors growth of *Acinetobacter*.[17]

Surveillance and Control of Pathogens of Epidemiological Importance Program

Data from the Surveillance and Control of Pathogens of Epidemiological Importance (SCOPE) program showed that *A baumannii* accounted for 86% of all *Acinetobacter* species identified from BSIs. Although the study found that *Acinetobacter*-caused BSIs represented only 1.3% of the

Occurrence by Site of Infection

Respiratory	Wound	Urine
1,659	633	651
2.0	2.2	0.2
(1.4-3.9)	(2.0-2.4)	(0.0-0.4)
6,711	2,191	2,569
2.5	2.1	1.0
(2.3-2.8)	(2.0-2.2)	(0.9-1.0)
1,914	1,353	1,430
9.7	4./	2.2
(7.1-11.6)	(3.5-5.5)	(0.9-3.2)

total BSIs, the crude mortality associated with BSIs caused by *Acinetobacter* was 43.4% among patients in ICUs.[9]

Wounds Among Military Personnel

Between January 1, 2002, and August 31, 2004, military health officials identified 102 patients with *A baumannii* at military medical facilities where service members received treatment for injuries sustained in Afghanistan, Iraq, and Kuwait.[18] At one facility, of 33 patients with *A baumannii* BSI, 30 (91%) had received traumatic injuries and were transferred to an ICU. In 22 (67%)

of those patients, BSI was detected from blood culture within 48 hours of ICU admission.

Of 45 patients with *A baumannii* BSI at another medical facility, 29 (64%) had sustained traumatic injuries. Of these, 18 (62%) had BSI detected from blood culture within 48 hours of hospital admission after transfer from a combat theater medical facility or other medical facility. At one medical facility, 13 (35%) of isolates were susceptible to imipenem only and 2 (4%) were resistant to all drugs tested.

Costs Associated With Acinetobacter *Infections*

Multidrug-resistant *Acinetobacter baumannii* (MDRAB) is a particular problem in hospital burn units, where patients are likely to have large, open wounds and are often on mechanical ventilation.[19] Wilson et al[19] analyzed the costs associated with *A baumannii* infections in the burn unit of a public teaching hospital over a period of 1 year. Results indicated that the mean total hospital cost for patients who acquired MDRAB while in the burn unit was $98,575 higher than that for the control group. The higher total cost was caused by increased length of stay as well as increased daily cost of care, involving longer and more expensive courses of antibiotics, repeat surgeries for failed skin grafts, and other complications.

Analysis of an increase in *A baumannii* infections in an ICU at another teaching hospital over a 1-year period showed increased cost caused by more use of ventilators than for patients with non-*Acinetobacter* cultures, longer length of stay, longer duration and greater number of antibiotics used, more bed transfers, and higher hospital and pharmacy charges.[20]

Control Measures

Colonization with *Acinetobacter* often precedes infection. Hand colonization can be controlled by proper handwashing, glove use, or use of alcohol-based antiseptics or soaps. Strict isolation of infected or colonized patients to limit transmission is an effective control measure.[21]

Table 5-4: Measures to Control Transmission of *Acinetobacter*

- Reduce colonization
  - Proper handwashing
  - Use of gloves
  - Use of alcohol-based antiseptics or soaps
  - Strict isolation of infected or colonized patients

- Disinfect environment
  - Disinfect infected/colonized patient after discharge
  - Disinfect reusable equipment

- Control use of antimicrobials to reduce selective pressure

- Temporarily close unit if other measures fail

High standards of cleanliness play an important role in reducing environmental contamination.[21] In some cases, temporary closure of the patient care unit for complete disinfection may be required.

Use of broad-spectrum antimicrobials has been proven to promote development of resistance. Controlling antimicrobial use, therefore, is an important part of preventive measures against emergence of MDRAB (Table 5-4).[22]

Clinical Infections

Acinetobacter species can cause a wide variety of clinical infections, including pneumonia, bacteremia, endocarditis, meningitis, urinary tract infections, skin and soft-tissue infections, and peritonitis.[5] Osteomyelitis and ophthalmic infections are uncommon.[5]

Bloodstream Infections

A baumannii BSIs are most commonly observed among patients in ICUs.[9] Antimicrobial resistance rates and associated mortality are high for *A baumannii* BSIs. Known

Table 5-5: Sources of Bloodstream Infection Caused by *Acinetobacter*

Source of entry	All *Acinetobacter* species (n = 129)
Intravenous device	26 (20.2)
Respiratory tract	21 (16.3)
Urinary tract	2 (1.6)
GI tract	3 (2.3)
Wound infection	7 (5.4)
Other	6 (4.6)
Unknown	64 (49.6)

BSI = bloodstream infection; GI = gastrointestinal
Adapted from Wisplinghoff et al, *Clin Infect Dis* 2000;31:690-697.

risk factors for *A baumannii* bacteremia include invasive procedures, use of broad-spectrum antibiotics,[23] and presence of surgical wounds and burns.[24] Intravenous (IV) catheter site infections and respiratory tract infections are common sources of bacteremia (Table 5-5).[25] Outbreaks of *Acinetobacter* sepsis in neonates have been reported in Japan, Israel, and India. Mean birth weight and previous antibiotic therapy were the primary factors associated with these neonatal infections.[26]

Endocarditis caused by *Acinetobacter* is uncommon, but cases of native-valve infective endocarditis have been

No. (%) of Patients With BSI Caused by		
Acinetobacter non-*baumannii* (n = 18)	*Acinetobacter baumannii* (n = 111)	Other gram-negative pathogens (n = 2,952)
2 (11.1)	24 (21.6)	470 (15.9)
1 (5.6)	20 (18)	324 (11.0)
—	2 (1.8)	462 (15.6)
1 (5.6)	2 (1.8)	190 (6.4)
2 (11.1)	5 (4.5)	152 (5.2)
2 (11.1)	4 (3.6)	114 (3.9)
10 (55.6)	54 (48.6)	240 (42.0)

reported.[27] Prior dental procedures and cardiac surgery have been associated with these infections.

Intra-abdominal Infections

Peritonitis associated with continuous ambulatory peritoneal dialysis has been reported, as have *Acinetobacter* infections associated with biliary stents and postoperative sites.[5]

Respiratory Tract Infections

The respiratory tract is a common site for *Acinetobacter* infection. Community-acquired *Acinetobacter* pneumonia usually occurs in patients with compromised host defenses caused by underlying conditions, such as alcoholism, smoking, diabetes mellitus, chronic obstructive pulmonary disease, and renal failure.[10,11]

However, *Acinetobacter* species have had the greatest impact as the cause of nosocomial pneumonia, particularly ventilator-associated pneumonia.[2] Ventilator-associated pneumonia occurs frequently in patients with severe underlying illnesses associated with prolonged hospital or ICU stay.[28] Predisposing factors for nosocomial *Acinetobacter* pneumonia include underlying pulmonary disease, endotracheal intubation, tracheostomy, recent surgery, ICU stay, and previous antibiotic therapy.[2] Complications may include septic shock and secondary bacteremia.

Skin and Soft Tissue Infections

Indwelling venous catheters are portals of entry for *Acinetobacter* infection, which may result in cellulitis.[2] Traumatic wounds, burns, and surgical incision sites may become colonized with *Acinetobacter* with resultant infection. While generally localized, complications from skin and soft-tissue infections may include bacteremia, especially in burn patients.[29]

Urinary Tract Infections

Acinetobacter species are rarely the cause of urinary tract infections, despite colonization of the urinary tract.[2] However, in the presence of nephrolithiasis or indwelling urinary catheters, *Acinetobacter* cystitis and pyelonephritis can develop.

Central Nervous System Infections

Meningitis caused by *Acinetobacter* also occurs infrequently[2] and is usually a postoperative complication after neurosurgery.[30] In one report, isolates cultured from suctioning equipment were shown to match the *A baumannii* strain involved in an outbreak.[28]

Treatment

Carbapenems

The rapid evolution of antimicrobial resistance has greatly reduced options for effective therapy for infections caused by *Acinetobacter* species. Carbapenems became the treatment of choice following *Acinetobacter* resistance to fluoroquinolones, aminoglycosides, and third-generation cephalosporins. Carbapenem resistance has, however, further reduced choices for treatment of resistant *Acinetobacter*.

Carbapenemases are β-lactamases that significantly hydrolyze at least imipenem and/or meropenem.[31] Carbapenemases of Ambler class B enzymes (metalloenzymes) are the most clinically significant carbapenemases. They hydrolyze virtually all β-lactams except aztreonam (Azactam®).[31] Carbapenemases of Ambler class D (oxacillinases) have less effect on susceptibility for imipenem and meropenem.

Previous use of antimicrobials, especially third-generation cephalosporins, has been linked to subsequent development of resistance in *Acinetobacter*. Landman et al analyzed a citywide outbreak of MDRAB in Brooklyn, New York, in 1998.[32] Their data indicated use of third-generation cephalosporins was associated with carbapenem resistance in *Acinetobacter*, which had been previously observed by other investigators.[33,34] Another study demonstrated that increased use of imipenem against cephalosporin-resistant *Klebsiella pneumoniae* promoted the development of imipenem-resistant *A baumannii*.[14]

Alternatives to Carbapenems

Alternatives to carbapenem use for treatment of MDRAB include colistin (Coly-Mycin® S) and polymyxin B (Aerosporin®) and various antimicrobial combinations (Table 5-6).[35,36] A Spanish study of 35 episodes of ventilator-associated *A baumannii* pneumonia treated with colistin yielded encouraging results.[35] Twenty-one patients had illness caused by a strain susceptible only to colistin; 14 patients' illness was caused by strains still susceptible to imipenem. Intravenous colistin clinically cured 57% of patients in both groups, with no sign of neuromuscular

Table 5-6: Antimicrobial Agents Frequently Active Against *Acinetobacter baumannii*

Single agents

- Imipenem
- Meropenem (Merrem®)
- Amikacin (Amikin®)
- Polymyxin B (Aerosporin®)
- Colistin (Coly-Mycin® S)
- Ampicillin/sulbactam (Unasyn®)

Synergistic or additive combinations (in vitro or mouse model)

- Polymyxin B plus rifampin (Rifadin®, Rimactane®), imipenem, meropenem, azithromycin (Zithromax®), or sulfamethoxazole/trimethoprim (Bactrim®, Cotrim®, Septra®, Sulfatrim®)
- Rifampin plus imipenem or tobramycin (Nebcin®)
- Imipenem plus an aminoglycoside
- Sulbactam plus fosfomycin (Monurol®)
- Fluoroquinolones plus β-lactams
- Fluoroquinolones plus amikacin (Amikin®)

blockade. The investigators concluded that IV colistin appeared to be safe and effective for ventilator-associated pneumonia caused by *A baumannii*.

Polymyxins

Colistin (polymyxin E) and polymyxin B are broad-spectrum antimicrobials originally used during the 1960s and 1970s. Both polymyxins are bactericidal. They target the bacterial cell wall and disrupt membrane permeability, which leads to the death of the bacteria. Colistin is available for parenteral administration as colistimethate (Coly-Mycin® M) and for topical or oral use as colistin sulfate. Colistin concentrates in the kidneys, muscle, liver, heart, and lungs and is primarily excreted via the kidneys. After nephrotoxic and neurotoxic adverse effects were observed, colistin was seldom prescribed. However, as MDRAB has emerged, there is renewed interest in colistin as an alternate therapy.

Falagas et al analyzed data for 19 courses of prolonged (more than 4 weeks) IV colistin.[37] The study observed no serious toxicity in the patients who received IV colistin therapy and concluded that colistin should be considered for treatment of multidrug-resistant gram-negative bacteria. Serum creatinine, blood urea, liver function tests, and signs and symptoms of neurotoxicity were the main outcomes studied. No apnea or evidence of neuromuscular blockade was found in this study. Another study compared treatment with IV colistin to treatment with imipenem/cilastatin for multidrug-resistant ventilator-associated pneumonia.[35] Results indicated comparable efficacy and no observable nephrotoxicity or neurotoxicity. In terms of clinical response, the outcome for patients treated with colistin did not differ from the outcome for patients treated with imipenem. The study recommended, however, that carbapenems should remain the antibiotics of choice for susceptible strains and that colistin may be an effective alternative for carbapenem-resistant strains.

Another study suggested that aerosolized colistin may be an effective adjunctive treatment for nosocomial pneumonia caused by multidrug-resistant gram-negative bacteria.[38] Investigators retrospectively reviewed the medical records of eight hospital patients who had received aerosolized colistin as adjunctive therapy for multidrug-resistant pneumonia. The daily dose of colistin ranged from 1.5 to 6 million IU divided into three or four doses, and mean duration of administration was 10.5 days. The pneumonia responded to treatment in seven of the eight patients, and no bronchoconstriction or chest tightness was reported. Aerosolized colistin has been used to treat or prevent lung infections in patients with cystic fibrosis, but additional studies are needed to confirm the effectiveness of nebulized colistin as an adjunct to IV antimicrobial treatment in patients without cystic fibrosis.

Reis et al reported that increased use of polymyxins for carbapenem-resistant *Acinetobacter* in Brazil resulted in emergence of polymyxin resistance.[39] In their study between September 1999 and December 2000, five *Acinetobacter* isolates with polymyxin resistance were identified in a tertiary care hospital in Brazil. Once again, emergence of resistance was likely caused by overuse of an agent, resulting in selective antimicrobial pressure.

Combination Therapy

Combination therapy is used to expand the antimicrobial spectrum, minimize toxicity, and reduce or prevent the emergence of resistant mutant bacterial strains.[40] Because emergence of resistant strains is a result of selective pressure induced by antimicrobial therapy, the chance of resistance to two classes of antimicrobials in the parent population is a product of mutation frequencies, as long as the mechanisms of resistance are different.[40]

Sulbactam is a β-lactamase inhibitor with activity against *Acinetobacter* species. Sulbactam binds to penicillin-binding protein 2, which accounts for its antibacterial activity. In the United States, sulbactam is available only in combination with ampicillin. It is widely distributed in the body, with the exception of poor penetration into the cerebrospinal fluid in patients without meningeal inflammation. Sulbactam is generally well tolerated and is excreted primarily unchanged in the urine.

Use of sulbactam against *Acinetobacter* species was first reported in 1993 for an outbreak of imipenem-resistant *Acinetobacter* in New York.[41] In vitro susceptibility testing indicated that ampicillin/sulbactam had the best activity against resistant *Acinetobacter* compared to amoxicillin/clavulanate (Augmentin®) and piperacillin/tazobactam (Zosyn®).

A retrospective analysis of 48 patients with *Acinetobacter* bacteremia in a university teaching hospital indicated that ampicillin/sulbactam was as effective as imipenem/cilastatin, based on clinical response at days 2 and 7 and at the end of treatment.[42] Bacteremia was eradicated in 97% of the patients receiving ampicillin/sulbactam and in 100% of the imipenem-treated patients.

Additional Combinations

Synergistic relationships between two or more antimicrobials used against *Acinetobacter* species have been documented in studies using a mouse model. These studies indicate enhanced effect for colistin and rifampin (Rifadin®, Rimactane®),[43] and in cases where rifampin resistance was only moderate, rifampin plus imipenem or rifampin plus tobramycin was effective.[36] In cases of moderate imipenem resistance, imipenem plus aminoglycosides was effective.

Manikal et al tested combinations of polymyxin B and other agents against *Acinetobacter* species and documented synergistic effects with polymyxin B and rifampin, meropenem, azithromycin, and sulfamethoxazole/trimethoprim.[44] A combination of sulbactam and fosfomycin also resulted in enhanced activity. Additional in vitro studies showed that polymyxin B plus imipenem or rifampin was effective against *Acinetobacter* isolates.[45] Eight *A baumanii* isolates resistant to all common antibiotics were exposed to polymyxin B, imipenem, and rifampin. Polymyxin with each of the other drugs was synergistic. Double combinations of polymyxin B and imipenem and polymyxin B and rifampin killed seven of the eight isolates, and triple combinations killed all isolates within a day.[45] An Italian study reported that combinations of fluoroquinolones with β-lactams or amikacin possessed enhanced activity against *Acinetobacter* species.[46] Levofloxacin (Levaquin®) and ciprofloxacin (Cipro®) combined with ceftazidime, as well as levofloxacin combined with amikacin, were synergistic for all strains of *Pseudomonas aeruginosa* and *Acinetobacter* tested.

Treatment with an effective antibiotic should be based on susceptibility patterns at the individual medical center. Clonally related strains of *Acinetobacter* that differ in susceptibility patterns may coexist within a single hospital, depending on the selective pressure related to antibiotic exposure in various areas.

Future Directions

A new class of antibiotics, the glycylcyclines, has been developed specifically to overcome the problem of tetracycline resistance.[47] Tigecycline (Tygacil™), a novel, broad-spectrum glycylcycline, is a minocycline derivative that shows high activity in vitro against *Acinetobacter* strains resistant to imipenem.[48,49] It is also effective in vitro against a broad range of gram-positive, gram-negative, atypical, anaerobic, and antibiotic-resistant bacteria.[49]

In clinical trials, tigecycline seems to have good efficacy and tolerability against many clinically relevant pathogens, including those resistant to tetracyclines.[49] It is only available as an IV preparation and seems to have good tissue penetration with potential for use for complicated skin and soft tissue infections and intra-abdominal infections. Because of its long half-life and post-antibiotic effect, once-daily dosing may be possible, but there is no data to support this use at time of publication. Tygacil™ received FDA approval in June 2005.

References

1. Gales AC, Jones RN, Forward KR, et al: Emerging importance of multidrug-resistant *Acinetobacter* species and Stenotrophomonas maltophilia as pathogens in seriously ill patients: geographic patterns, epidemiological features, and trends in the SENTRY Antimicrobial Surveillance Program (1997-1999). *Clin Infect Dis* 2001;32(suppl 2):S104-S113.

2.   Allen DM, Hartman BJ: *Acinetobacter* species. In: *Mandell, Douglas, and Bennett's Principles and Practice of Infectious Diseases.* 5th ed. Philadelphia, PA, Churchill Livingstone, 2000, pp 2009-2012.

3.   Pier GB: Molecular mechanisms of microbial pathogenesis. In: Braunwald E, Fauci AS, Kasper DL, et al, eds. *Harrison's Principles of Internal Medicine,* 15th ed. New York, NY, McGraw-Hill, 2001, pp 767-774.

4.   Jain R, Danziger LH: Multidrug-resistant *Acinetobacter* infections: an emerging challenge to clinicians. *Ann Pharmacother* 2004;38:1449-1459.

5.   Russo TA: Diseases caused by gram-negative enteric bacilli. In: Braunwald E, Fauci AS, Kasper DL, et al, eds. *Harrison's Principles of Internal Medicine.* 15th ed. New York, NY, McGraw-Hill, 2001, pp 953-960.

6.   Bergogne-Bérézin E, Towner KJ: *Acinetobacter* spp. as nosocomial pathogens: microbiological, clinical, and epidemiological features. *Clin Microbiol Rev* 1996;9:148-165.

7.   Henrichsen J, Blom J: Correlation between twitching motility and possession of polar fimbriae in *Acinetobacter calcoaceticus. Acta Pathol Microbiol Scand* 1975;83:103-115.

8.   Poh CL, Loh GK: Enzymatic profile of clinical isolates of *Acinetobacter calcoaceticus. Med Microbiol Immunol (Berl)* 1985;174:29-33.

9.   Wisplinghoff H, Bischoff T, Tallent SM, et al: Nosocomial bloodstream infections in US hospitals: analysis of 24,179 cases from a prospective nationwide surveillance study. *Clin Infect Dis* 2004;39:309-317.

10.   Anstey NM, Currie BJ, Withnall KM: Community-acquired *Acinetobacter pneumonia* in the Northern Territory of Australia. *Clin Infect Dis* 1992;14:83-91.

11.   Goodhart GL, Abrutyn E, Watson R, et al: Community-acquired *Acinetobacter calcoaceticus* var anitratus pneumonia. *JAMA* 1977;238:1516-1518.

12.   Larson EL: Persistent carriage of gram-negative bacteria on hands. *Am J Infect Control* 1981;9:112-119.

13.   Allen KD, Green HT: Hospital outbreak of multi-resistant *Acinetobacter anitratus*: an airborne mode of spread? *J Hosp Infect* 1987;9:110-119.

14.   Go ES, Urban C, Burns J, et al: Clinical and molecular epidemiology of *Acinetobacter* infections sensitive only to polymyxin B and sulbactam. *Lancet* 1994;344:1329-1332.

15.   Mahgoub S, Ahmed J, Glatt AE: Underlying characteristics of patients harboring highly resistant *Acinetobacter baumannii*. *Am J Infect Control* 2002;30:386-390.

16.   National Nosocomial Infection Surveillance (NNIS) System report, data summary from October 1986-April 1998, issued June 1998. *Am J Infect Control* 1998;26:522-533.

17.   McDonald LC, Banerjee SN, Jarvis WR: Seasonal variation of *Acinetobacter* infections: 1987-1996. National Nosocomial Infection Surveillance System. *Clin Infect Dis* 1999;29:1133-1137.

18.   Centers for Disease Control and Prevention: *Acinetobacter baumannii* infections among patients at military medical facilities treating injured U.S. service members, 2002-2004. *MMWR Morb Mortal Wkly Rep* 2004;53:1063-1066.

19.   Wilson SJ, Knipe CJ, Zieger MJ, et al: Direct costs of multidrug-resistant *Acinetobacter baumannii* in the burn unit of a public teaching hospital. *Am J Infect Control* 2004;32:342-344.

20.   Weingarten CM, Rybak MJ, Jahns BE, et al: Evaluation of *Acinetobacter baumannii* infections and colonization, and antimicrobial treatment patterns in an urban teaching hospital. *Pharmacotherapy* 1999;19:1080-1085.

21.   Simor AE, Lee M, Vearncombe M, et al: An outbreak due to multiresistant *Acinetobacter baumannii* in a burn unit: risk factors for acquisition and management. *Infect Control Hosp Epidemiol* 2002;23:261-267.

22.   Urban C, Segal-Maurer S, Rahal JJ: Considerations in control and treatment of nosocomial infections due to multidrug-resistant *Acinetobacter baumannii*. *Clin Infect Dis* 2003;36:1268-1274.

23.   Cisneros JM, Rodriguez-Bano J: Nosocomial bacteremia due to *Acinetobacter baumannii*: epidemiology, clinical features, and treatment. *Clin Microbiol Infect* 2002;8:687-693.

24.   Wisplinghoff H, Perbix W, Seifert H: Risk factors for nosocomial bloodstream infections due to *Acinetobacter baumannii*: a case-control study of adult burn patients. *Clin Infect Dis* 1999;28:59-66.

25.   Wisplinghoff H, Edmond MB, Pfaller MA, et al: Nosocomial bloodstream infections caused by *Acinetobacter* species in United

States hospitals: clinical features, molecular epidemiology, and antimicrobial susceptibility. *Clin Infect Dis* 2000;31:690-697.

26. Sakata H, Fujita K, Maruyama S, et al: *Acinetobacter calcoaceticus* biovar anitratus septicaemia in a neonatal intensive care unit: epidemiology and control. *J Hosp Infect* 1989;14:15-22.

27. Gradon JD, Chapnick EK, Lutwick LI: Infective endocarditis of a native valve due to *Acinetobacter*: case report and review. *Clin Infect Dis* 1992;14:1145-1148.

28. Wood GC, Hanes SD, Croce MA, et al: Comparison of ampicillin-sulbactam and imipenem-cilastatin for the treatment of *Acinetobacter* ventilator-associated pneumonia. *Clin Infect Dis* 2002;34:1425-1430.

29. Tilley PA, Roberts FJ: Bacteremia with *Acinetobacter* species: risk factors and prognosis in different clinical settings. *Clin Infect Dis* 1994;18:896-900.

30. Wroblewska MM, Dijkshoorn L, Marchel H, et al: Outbreak of nosocomial meningitis caused by *Acinetobacter baumannii* in neurosurgical patients. *J Hosp Infect* 2004;57:300-307.

31. Nordmann P, Poirel L: Emerging carbapenemases in gram-negative aerobes. *Clin Microbiol Infect* 2002;8:321-331.

32. Landman D, Quale JM, Mayorga D, et al: Citywide clonal outbreak of multiresistant *Acinetobacter baumannii* and *Pseudomonas aeruginosa* in Brooklyn, NY: the preantibiotic era has returned. *Arch Intern Med* 2002;162:1515-1520.

33. Mulin B, Talon D, Viel JF, et al: Risk factors for nosocomial colonization with multiresistant *Acinetobacter baumannii*. *Eur J Clin Microbiol Infect Dis* 1995;14:569-576.

34. Scerpella EG, Wanger AR, Armitige L, et al: Nosocomial outbreak caused by a multiresistant clone of *Acinetobacter baumannii*: results of the case-control and molecular epidemiologic investigations. *Infect Control Hosp Epidemiol* 1995;16:92-97.

35. Garnacho-Montero J, Ortiz-Leyba C, Jiménez-Jiménez FJ, et al: Treatment of multidrug-resistant *Acinetobacter baumannii* ventilator-associated pneumonia (VAP) with intravenous colistin: a comparison with imipenem-susceptible VAP. *Clin Infect Dis* 2003;36:1111-1118.

36. Montero A, Ariza J, Corbella X, et al: Antibiotic combinations for serious infections caused by carbapenem-resistant *Acinetobacter baumannii* in a mouse pneumonia model. *J Antimicrob Chemother* 2004;54:1085-1091.

37. Falagas ME, Rizos M, Bliziotis IA, et al: Toxicity after prolonged (more than four weeks) administration of intravenous colistin. *BMC Infect Dis* 2005;5:1.

38. Michalopoulos A, Kasiakou S, Mastora Z, et al: Aerosolized colistin for the treatment of nosocomial pneumonia due to multidrug-resistant gram-negative bacteria in patients without cystic fibrosis. *Critical Care* 2005;9:R53-R59.

39. Reis AO, Luz DA, Tognim MC, et al: Polymyxin-resistant *Acinetobacter* spp. isolates: what is next? *Emerg Infect Dis* 2003;9:1025-1027.

40. Mouton JW: Combination therapy as a tool to prevent emergence of bacterial resistance. *Infection* 1999;27(suppl 2):S24-S28.

41. Urban C, Go E, Mariano N, et al: Effect of sulbactam on infection caused by imipenem-resistant *Acinetobacter calcoaceticus* biotype anitratus. *J Infect Dis* 1993;167:448-451.

42. Jellison TK, Mckinnon PS, Rybak MJ: Epidemiology, resistance, and outcomes of *Acinetobacter baumannii* bacteremia treated with imipenem-cilastatin or ampicillin-sulbactam. *Pharmacotherapy* 2001;21:142-148.

43. Wolff M, Joly-Guillou ML, Farinotti R, et al: In vivo efficacies of combinations of β-lactams, β-lactamase inhibitors, and rifampin against *Acinetobacter baumannii* in a mouse pneumonia model. *Antimicrob Agents Chemother* 1999;43:1406-1411.

44. Manikal VM, Landman D, Saurina G, et al: Endemic carbapenem-resistant *Acinetobacter* species in Brooklyn, New York: citywide prevalence, interinstitutional spread, and relation to antibiotic usage. *Clin Infect Dis* 2000;31:101-106.

45. Yoon J, Urban C, Terzian C, et al: In vitro double and triple synergistic activities of polymyxin B, imipenem, and rifampin against multidrug-resistant *Acinetobacter baumannii*. *Antimicrob Agents Chemother* 2004;48:753-757.

46. Drago L, De Vecchi E, Nicola L, et al: Activity of levofloxacin and ciprofloxacin in combination with cefepime, ceftazidime, imipenem, piperacillin-tazobactam, and amikacin against different *Pseudomonas aeruginosa* phenotypes and *Acinetobacter* spp. *Chemotherapy* 2004;50:202-210.

47. Petersen PJ, Jacobus NV, Weiss WJ, et al: In vitro and in vivo antibacterial activities of a new glycylcycline, the 9-t-butylglycylamido derivative of minocycline (GAR-936). *Antimicrob Agents Chemother* 1999;43:738-744.

48. Pachón-Ibáñez ME, Jiménez-Mejías ME, Pichardo C, et al: Activity of tigecycline (GAR-936) against *Acinetobacter baumannii* strains, including those resistant to imipenem. *Antimicrob Agents Chemother* 2004;48:4479-4481.

49. Milatovic D, Schmitz FJ, Verhoef J, et al: Activities of the glycylcycline tigecycline (GAR-936) against 1,924 recent European clinical bacterial isolates. *Antimicrob Agents Chemother* 2003;47:400-404.

 Chapter **6**

Enterobacter

E *nterobacter* species are normal commensals of the gastrointestinal (GI) tract and seldom cause infections in healthy individuals.[1] However, similar to most other members of the Enterobacteriaceae family, they can be responsible for opportunistic infections in immunocompromised or debilitated patients.

Enterobacter are among the most common gram-negative pathogens found in the hospital. They cause 5% to 7% of cases of nosocomial bacteremia[2] and are associated with relatively high mortality rates.[3,4] Although the organisms are primarily associated with health-care facilities, strains have also been implicated in community-acquired infections.[5] Because most *Enterobacter* are resistant to older antibiotics and can rapidly develop resistance to newer antimicrobials during therapy, options for effective treatment are increasingly limited.

Clinical Microbiology

Enterobacter are gram-negative bacteria that can cause a broad range of clinical infections, including bacteremia and infections of the respiratory tract, urinary tract, GI tract, skin and soft tissues, bones and joints, and central nervous system.[5]

There are at least 14 *Enterobacter* species, but *E cloacae* and *E aerogenes* account for most infections (65% to 75%, and 15% to 25%, respectively).[5,6] Other *Enterobacter* that cause infections in humans include *E agglomerans* (5%), which has been renamed *Pantoea agglomerans*;

E sakazakii (1%); and *E gergoviae* (<1%). Because antimicrobial susceptibility varies widely among the species of *Enterobacter*, laboratory analysis for identification of the species is an important key to selection of appropriate therapy.[5]

Enterobacter are prevalent in food, in various animals, and on environmental surfaces, including medical equipment.[7] *E sakazakii* is particularly resistant to drying and osmotic stresses when its cells are in a stationary phase.[8]

Antimicrobial Resistance

Enterobacter exhibit intrinsic resistance to many antimicrobials, including ampicillin and first- and second-generation cephalosporins,[5,7] (Table 6-1).[9] In addition, the use of β-lactam antibiotics may result in rapid development of resistance during therapy.[5-7]

Extensive use of third-generation cephalosporins, such as cefotaxime (Claforan®), ceftazidime (Ceptaz®, Fortaz®), and ceftriaxone (Rocephin®), has resulted in the emergence of derepressed mutant *Enterobacter* strains.[7,10,11] These strains produce high levels of the chromosomal AmpC cephalosporinase and confer resistance to extended-spectrum β-lactam antibiotics and aztreonam (Azactam®). These enzymes are called extended-spectrum β-lactamases (ESBLs).[7,10,11] Bacteria possessing ESBLs are also often resistant to β-lactam/β-lactamase inhibitor combinations, such as ticarcillin/clavulanate (Timentin®) and piperacillin/tazobactam (Zosyn®).[3,5,7,10-12]

Kaye et al reported that approximately 19% of patients treated with cephalosporins will develop resistance.[10] Their study also indicated that while broad-spectrum cephalosporins were associated with the emergence of *Enterobacter* resistance to those agents, exposure to narrow- and expanded-spectrum cephalosporins was not associated with the emergence of such resistance. In addition, isolates from patients with *Enterobacter* bacteremia showed higher rates of emerging resistance than did isolates from patients with tissue, wound, or urinary infections.

Table 6-1: In Vitro Antimicrobial Agent Susceptibilities of *E aerogenes* and *E cloacae*

Antimicrobial agent	E aerogenes		E cloacae	
	% resistant			
	ICU	Non-ICU	ICU	Non-ICU
Amikacin	0.9	1.3	0.9	0.5
Ampicillin/ sulbactam	58.8	49.4	71.4	65.6
Cefepime	10.4	1.0	5.9	3.8
Cefotaxime	15.7	16.9	33.9	25.3
Ceftazidime	34.6	22.9	37.0	28.9
Ceftriaxone	11.8	6.2	28.9	23.0
Ciprofloxacin	5.9	5.6	8.6	8.9
Gentamicin	7.4	3.4	8.7	7.8
Imipenem	0	0	0	0
Levofloxacin	3.3	4.4	9.1	8.3
Meropenem	0.5	0	0	0
Piperacillin/ tazobactam	8.9	8.9	21.8	18.9
Ticarcillin/ clavulanate	33.4	22.1	37.5	27.1
Trimethoprim/ sulfamethoxazole	3.7	5.0	11.6	12.0

Adapted from Karlowsky[9] data from The Surveillance Network (1998-2001).

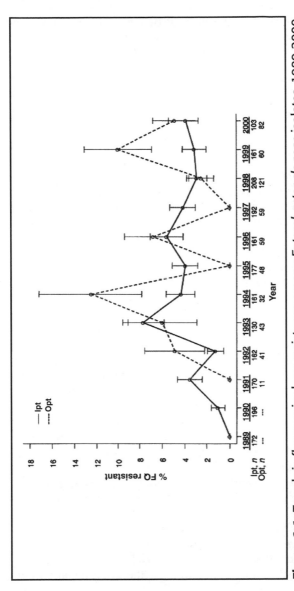

Figure 6-1: Trends in fluoroquinolone resistance among *Enterobacter cloacae* isolates, 1989-2000. FQ, fluoroquinolone; Ipt, isolates obtained from inpatients; Opt, isolates obtained from outpatients. Bars show 95% confidence intervals (CIs) From Lautenbach.[14]

A study by Kang et al of patients with *Enterobacter* bacteremia found that ciprofloxacin (Cipro®) resistance was closely associated with prior use of fluoroquinolones and broad-spectrum cephalosporin resistance.[13]

Lautenbach et al tracked trends in fluoroquinolone resistance among Enterobacteriaceae isolates during a 12-year period.[14] The study showed that fluoroquinolone resistance varies between inpatient and outpatient populations and between *Enterobacter* species (Figures 6-1 and 6-2).

Mechanisms of Resistance

Enterobacter have two main mechanisms of antimicrobial resistance: production of an inactivating enzyme, and alteration of the ability of a drug to enter and/or accumulate in the cell.[5]

In some *Enterobacter* strains, such as *E agglomerans*, *E gergoviae*, and some *E sakazakii*, β-lactamase is produced at low, noninducible levels, and these species remain susceptible to most β-lactam antimicrobials. In *E aerogenes*, *E cloacae*, and most *E sakazakii*, however, the production of inducible β-lactamase results in greater hydrolysis of the drug and, therefore, in greater resistance.[5]

In addition to β-lactamases, *Enterobacter* have been reported to produce chromosomally encoded carbapenemase, resulting in carbapenem resistance[15] and aminoglycoside-inactivating enzymes conferring aminoglycoside resistance.[16,17]

Extended-spectrum β-lactamases (ESBLs) were discovered in Europe in the 1980s after widespread use of broad-spectrum antibiotics.[18] In addition to often conferring resistance to extended-spectrum antibiotics, ESBL genes can transfer to other bacterial species on plasmids, especially in hospitals and long-term-care facilities, further limiting choices for antimicrobial therapy.[18,19]

Porins and Efflux Pumps

Bacterial porins are proteins that form water-filled channels in the outer membrane of the gram-negative cell.

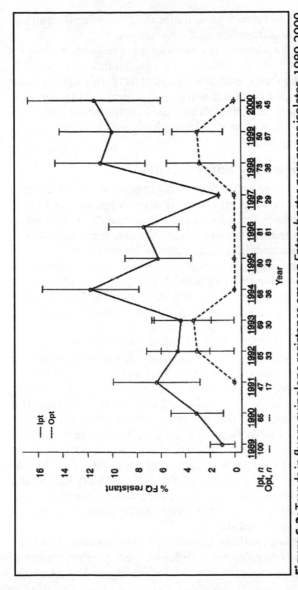

Figure 6-2: Trends in fluoroquinolone resistance among *Enterobacter aerogenes* isolates, 1989-2000. FQ, fluoroquinolone; Ipt, isolates obtained from inpatients; Opt, isolates obtained from outpatients. Bars show 95% confidence intervals (CIs). From Lautenbach.[14]

Porins allow small polar molecules, amino acids, and nutrients to diffuse across the membrane.

An efflux system is a mechanism of resistance whereby the bacterial cell actively pumps antibiotics out of the cell, reducing their concentration and effect on the cell. In some multidrug-resistant *E aerogenes*, a decrease in porin synthesis and an active efflux pump confer resistance to β-lactams, quinolones, chloramphenicol (Chloromycetin®), and imipenem.[20]

Pathogenicity and Virulence

Enterobacter are opportunistic organisms and are generally not virulent. Normal host defenses, including complement and phagocytosis, are usually sufficient in healthy individuals to prevent infection, but immunocompromised and debilitated patients are at risk.

Colonization is a major contributor to infection with *Enterobacter*.[7,21] Only a small percentage of individuals in the community are colonized, but the number of colonized patients increases significantly among hospitalized patients or those in long-term care facilities.[7]

Enterobacter infection appears to be a two-step process in which the host first acquires nosocomial flora, and then becomes infected from this carrier site.[22] Studies indicate that endogenous *Enterobacter* generally become pathogenic under broad-spectrum antibiotic therapy and are horizontally transmitted less often. Once in or on the host, bacterial adhesions and pili facilitate adhesion to host cells in most pathogens. Other virulence factors are those attributable to gram-negative bacteria in general. The lipopolysaccharide layer of the cellular outer membrane contains lipid A, an endotoxin that causes the manifestations of sepsis (fever, muscle proteolysis, intravascular coagulation, and shock).

Although little is known about the specific virulence factors of *Enterobacter*, different species exhibit features that enhance their potential for infection. For example,

E aerogenes and *E cloacae* have a greater resistance to disinfectants and antimicrobial agents than do other members of the Enterobacteriaceae family, which likely explains their predominance in hospitals.[23] *E cloacae* can also grow in 5% dextrose solution.

E sakazakii is associated with foodborne diseases causing meningitis or enteritis, especially in neonates and infants.[8] *E sakazakii* is resistant to desiccation and is able to grow on infant-feeding equipment and at refrigeration temperatures.[24,25]

E agglomerans also grows at low temperatures, is often associated with plants, and can be recovered from cotton.[26] *E agglomerans* has been implicated in outbreaks from contaminated intravenous (IV) solutions and in stored blood products.[27] It has also been found to cause 'cotton fever,' an acute febrile illness experienced by IV drug users who filter heroin through cotton before injection.[26]

Epidemiology

Enterobacter have become important nosocomial pathogens in many countries, and the emergence of antibiotic-resistant strains is of great concern.[21, 28-30] Members of the Enterobacteriaceae family comprise about 80% of gram-negative bacteria and 50% of all isolates identified in US hospitals.[31]

In 1997, the SENTRY Antimicrobial Surveillance Program documented bloodstream infections (BSIs) in a total of 4,267 nosocomial and community-acquired isolates from hospitals in the United States, Canada, and Latin America. *Enterobacter* species accounted for 9.4% of the isolates.[32]

The Surveillance Network (TSN) reported the prevalence of coresistant BSIs from ICU and non-ICU inpatient isolates among Enterobacteriaceae from 1998 to 2001. Table 6-1 shows the rates of resistance to extended-spectrum cephalosporins, other β-lactam antibiotics, and combinations of β-lactams and β-lactam inhibitors.[9]

Data from the Surveillance and Control of Pathogens of Epidemiological Importance (SCOPE) study of nosocomial BSIs in US hospitals showed a crude mortality rate of 32.5% for ICU patients with *Enterobacter* BSIs and 18% for non-ICU hospital patients.[3]

According to the National Nosocomial Infections Surveillance (NNIS) system report, *Enterobacter* species resistant to third-generation cephalosporins rank as the fourth most common nosocomial pathogens in ICUs.[33]

Although *Enterobacter* infections can be acquired from either endogenous or exogenous sources, it is likely that most nosocomial infections arise from colonized sites within the patient. Exogenous sources that have been identified include human and animal feces, water, plants, and dairy products. Single-source outbreaks have been attributed to contaminated IV solutions, blood products, powdered milk and infant formula, endoscopes, devices for monitoring intra-arterial pressure, and hands of personnel.[8,23,25,27]

Patients at greatest risk for *Enterobacter* infections are those who have severe underlying illness, experience prolonged hospital or ICU stay, and have received prior antibiotic therapy.[5,7] Immunosuppression, extremes of age, and the presence of a foreign device are additional risk factors.[5]

Costs

A study at Johns Hopkins Hospital evaluated the clinical and economic impact of the emergence of resistant *Enterobacter* species.[34] Patients with *Enterobacter* infections who developed resistance to third-generation cephalosporins were matched to control patients with *Enterobacter* infections who did not develop resistance. Twenty-six percent of those with resistance died vs 13% of control patients. The median hospital stay was 29.5 days for those with resistance and 19 days for controls, and hospital charges were $79,323 and $40,406 respectively. The study concluded that emergent antibiotic resistance in *Enterobacter* species results in increased mortality, length-of-stay, and hospital costs.

A retrospective, matched-cohort study by Blot et al compared ICU patients with nosocomial *Enterobacter* bacteremia to control patients without *Enterobacter*-caused bacteremia. They found no difference in mortality between case and control patients if effective antibiotic therapy was initiated promptly.[35]

Prevention

Because most *Enterobacter* infections arise from endogenous sources in colonized patients, the usual infection control measures of cohorting and screening patients are not likely to affect the overall incidence of this pathogen.[5] Restricting use of extended-spectrum cephalosporins, however, is recommended by a number of studies.[5,6,36]

For neonates, strict aseptic technique in the preparation of parenteral nutrition is recommended to reduce the risk of *Enterobacter* contamination,[1] and use of alcohol-based hand rubs is an alternative method to conventional handwashing in the hospital.[37]

Clinical Infections

Enterobacter species can cause various clinical infections, including bacteremia, respiratory tract infections, surgical and wound-site infections, intra-abdominal infections, and urinary tract infections.[3,5-7,38] *Enterobacter* endocarditis, meningitis, bone and joint infections, and ophthalmic infections are less common.[5,7,39]

Bloodstream infections (BSIs) are a major cause of morbidity and mortality.[3,5] Most bacteremias are nosocomial and occur most often in neonates and the elderly.[5] In a review of *Enterobacter* by Sanders and Sanders, *E cloacae* was found to be the predominate cause of nosocomial *Enterobacter* bacteremia (46% to 91% of isolates), followed by *E aerogenes* (9% to 43%), *E agglomerans*, *E sakazakii*, and others.[5] Of bacteremias involving *Enterobacter* species, 14% to 53% are polymicrobial.

Fever and rigors occur in up to 75% of patients with *Enterobacter* bacteremia and may appear in as short as 2 hours after infection of the bloodstream to as long as 20 days.[5] Additional manifestations of bacteremia may include hypotension,[6] altered mentation,[6] and both leukocytosis and leukopenia.

Severe underlying illness is the greatest risk factor for development of bacteremia,[5] and previous antimicrobial therapy, especially third-generation cephalosporin use, is another predisposing factor.[5-7] Other factors associated with *Enterobacter* bacteremia include diabetes mellitus, malignancy, cardiovascular disease, gastrointestinal diseases, burns, surgery, and previous *Enterobacter* infection. Intravascular catheters and urinary catheters are frequent sites for *Enterobacter* infection and subsequent bacteremia.[5,29]

Crude mortality rates for *Enterobacter* bacteremia range from 15% to 87%, with the highest rates occurring in transplant and burn units.[5]

Enterobacter endocarditis occurs infrequently and primarily affects individuals with abnormal native or prosthetic valves and IV drug abusers.[7,40] Underlying heart disease and IV drug abuse are major risk factors.

Meningitis caused by *Enterobacter* species is uncommon.[39,41] A review of data from the National Institute of Child Health and Human Development Neonatal Research Network identified only one case of *E sakazakii* meningitis/septicemia among 10,660 neonates.[39]

E sakazakii has, however, been implicated in a severe form of neonatal meningitis. Willis and Robinson found a 50% fatality rate in their study.[42] Contaminated infant formula has been identified as a source of infection in outbreaks and sporadic cases.[7,42] Complications of neonatal meningitis caused by *E sakazakii* include brain abscesses or cysts.[7,42]

Parodi et al described risk factors for *Enterobacter* meningitis in patients ≥18 years of age, during an 8-year period at a tertiary-care medical center.[43] External cerebral-spinal-fluid (CSF) drainage catheters, colonization or infection at non-CSF sites, and selective antimicrobial pressure were independent risk factors. Additional risk factors included advanced age, immunosuppression, and neurosurgery.

Enterobacter often cause intra-abdominal infections, partly because they are part of the normal flora of the GI tract.[5] *Enterobacter* may enter the peritoneum and viscera postoperatively, through perforation or by translocation.[5,7] Biliary stents are a known source of *Enterobacter* infection.[7]

Clinical manifestations of lower respiratory tract infections caused by *Enterobacter* include purulent bronchitis, pneumonia, lung abscess, and empyema, as well as asymptomatic colonization of respiratory secretions.[44] Nosocomial pneumonia is the leading cause of death in patients with hospital-acquired infections,[45] and the second most frequent cause of nosocomial infections.[46] Unless there is an extrapulmonary focus of *Enterobacter* infection, it is assumed *Enterobacter* pneumonia arises from normal flora that colonizes oropharyngeal secretions. Mortality associated with pneumonia may be as high as 50%,[5] and inadequate initial antimicrobial therapy is an independent risk factor for increased mortality (Table 6-2).[45,47,48]

Enterobacter species have also been associated with acute bacterial pneumonia in lung transplant recipients.[49] Although *S aureus* is the most common pathogen in donor lungs, *Enterobacter* species cause a greater percentage of pneumonia after transplantation (60% to 67%), while *S aureus* causes 12% to 27%.[49]

Enterobacter species can cause a range of skin and soft tissue infections, such as cellulitis, wound infections, and abscesses.[50,51] Jarvis et al analyzed data from the NNIS system and identified *Enterobacter* as one of the pathogens most commonly found in surgical wound infections.[52] Factors contributing to the outbreak included colonization of the sternum, groin, and wounds both before and after surgery, prophylactic use of cephalosporins, and co-infection with staphylococci in 25% of the patients.

Table 6-2: Risk Factors for the Development of Nosocomial Pneumonia

- Mechanical ventilation >48 hours
- Prior antibiotic use and resistance in ICU
- Duration of ICU or hospital stay
- Severity of underlying illness
- Acute respiratory distress syndrome, other health problems

Adapted from Lynch[48]

Enterobacter infections also occur in the community in previously healthy individuals.

Results from the SENTRY Antimicrobial Surveillance Program (2000) indicate *Enterobacter* are one of the top seven pathogens causing urinary tract infections, accounting for 4% of all isolates.[38] The incidence of *Enterobacter* among nosocomial urinary tract infections appears to be slowly increasing.[52]

Enterobacter cause only a small number of cases of postoperative endophthalmitis. But because the organism is aggressive and frequently multidrug resistant, *Enterobacter* postoperative endophthalmitis carries a poor prognosis.[53]

'Cotton Fever'

Ferguson et al identified *E agglomerans* as the causative agent in 'cotton fever,' a benign febrile illness seen in intravenous drug users.[26] Cotton and cotton plants are heavily colonized with *E agglomerans*, and heroin users who use cotton to filter the drug are at risk for this infection.

Treatment

The rise in multidrug-resistant gram-negative bacilli, including *Enterobacter* species, has limited therapeutic

Table 6-3: Third-generation Cephalosporins

- Cefdinir
- Cefixime
- Cefoperazone
- Cefotaxime
- Ceftazidime
- Ceftibuten
- Ceftizoxime
- Ceftriaxone
- Cefpodoxime

options for these opportunistic pathogens. *Enterobacter* exhibit chromosomally-mediated resistance to β-lactam antibiotics through production of AmpC β-lactamase enzymes.[54] And as new β-lactam antibiotics are developed to resist hydrolytic action of the enzymes, new β-lactamases emerge, causing resistance to each new drug. An example of this process is the third-generation extended-spectrum cephalosporins, which were widely used in the 1980s against serious gram-negative infections[55] (Table 6-3). Extended-spectrum β-lactamases (ESBLs) emerged with third-generation cephalosporin use. These enzymes are encoded on plasmids and readily transfer between species. More than 150 different ESBLs have been described,[55] and only carbapenems are reliably effective against organisms that produce ESBLs.[56]

In general, antimicrobials of first choice for treatment of *Enterobacter* infections include carbapenems and trimethoprim/sulfamethoxazole (TMP/SMX) (Bactrim®, Septra®), as well as aminoglycosides, cefepime (Maxipime®), and fluoroquinolones.[7,9,57] Table 6-4 lists suggestions for empiric antimicrobial therapy for serious *Enterobacter* infections and alternatives. The choice of empiric antibiotics for serious infections should be based on the pathogens and their susceptibility patterns in the institution where treatment is administered.

Table 6-4: Antimicrobial Therapy for *Enterobacter* Infections

Empiric Choices

- Imipenem
- Meropenem
- Cefepime
- Piperacillin/tazobactam
- Aminoglycoside
- Aztreonam
- Ciprofloxacin

Alternatives

- Trimethoprim/sulfamethoxazole
- Ticarcillin/clavulanate*
- Third-generation cephalosporin
- Levofloxacin

*For urinary tract infections only

Bloodstream infections are associated with significant morbidity and mortality, making appropriate initial antimicrobial therapy critical.[4] Studies by Setia and Gross showed that bacteremia-related mortality was reduced from 64% to 19% when antibiotic therapy was used that was active against the infecting organism.[58] In a similar study by Weinstein et al, mortality was three times lower when appropriate antibiotics were given.[59]

General management of bacteremia includes stopping or decreasing immunosuppressive medication and identifying the source of the bacteremia, if possible. If the source is an IV line, it should be removed, and if there is an abscess, it should be drained. Fluid replacement is important, as is maintenance of blood pressure. Antimicrobial therapy should be given as soon as the diagnosis is suspected.[60]

Data from the SENTRY Antimicrobial Surveillance Program indicate meropenem (Merrem®), imipenem

(Primaxin®), and cefepime (Maxipime®) are the most active antimicrobials against bloodstream infections for all gram-negative isolates, including *Enterobacter* species.[32] Aminoglycosides and fluoroquinolones tested were also active against *Enterobacter* isolates (Table 6-5).[61] In an 8-year study of antimicrobial susceptibilities to ESBL-producing strains of *Enterobacter*, Pai et al indicated that a confirmatory test for ESBL is necessary to use cefepime safely.[62]

In vitro studies indicate combination therapy may also be effective, using aztreonam plus a fluoroquinolone.[63] Critchley et al found aztreonam plus ciprofloxacin demonstrated synergy against 16.7% of gram-negative isolates in vitro. Ciprofloxacin resistance, however, has been reported in *Enterobacter* species causing bacteremia and is closely associated with broad-spectrum cephalosporin resistance and prior use of fluoroquinolones.[13]

Other investigators have suggested additional antimicrobial combinations, including cefepime plus ampicillin/sulbactam (Unasyn®),[64] a β-lactam plus an aminoglycoside or a fluoroquinolone, and moxifloxacin (Avelox®) plus either cefepime or piperacillin/tazobactam.[65]

Gram-negative organisms account for a small percentage of endocarditis. Gram-negative endocarditis generally occurs within the first 2 months after valve replacement in patients with prosthetic valves, caused by colonization by bacteria during bacteremia.[60] In general, empiric treatment while cultures are pending includes a combination of IV vancomycin (Vancocin®) and gentamicin (Garamycin®) plus rifampin (Rifadin®, Rimactane®). If *Enterobacter* is isolated, an aminoglycoside plus cefepime or a third-generation cephalosporin is suggested.

Careful asepsis and prompt removal of invasive devices are important measures for preventing postoperative infections in neurosurgical patients. Empiric therapy should be initiated for meningitis, followed by a cerebralspinal fluid examination within 30 minutes to identify the pathogen. Cefepime (or ceftazidime, if susceptible) plus gen-

Table 6-5: Susceptibilities of Most Active Antimicrobial Agents Against *Enterobacter* Bloodstream Isolates

Antimicrobial class and agent	% susceptible
β-lactam antimicrobial agents	
Cephalosporins (fourth-generation)	
• Cefepime	99.3
Carbapenems	
• Imipenem	98.6
• Meropenem	99.3
Non-β-lactam antimicrobial agents	
Aminoglycosides	
• Amikacin	100
• Gentamicin	94.3
• Tobramycin	93.9
Fluoroquinolones	
• Ciprofloxacin	92.2
• Ofloxacin	91.2
• Levofloxacin	93.2
Others	
• Trimethoprim/ sulfamethoxazole	84.4

Adapted from Pfaller[61] data from the SENTRY antimicrobial surveillance program tamicin is the suggested therapy for gram-negative bacilli, with IV ciprofloxacin and meropenem as alternatives.

A study of adult patients with postneurosurgical *Enterobacter* meningitis during an 8-year period evaluated risk factors, management, and treatment outcomes.[43] Parodi et al found TMP/SMX and carbapenems to be the most effective agents. Dosage adjustment is necessary with carbapenem use in patients with renal insufficiency to reduce the risk of seizures, especially in neurosurgical patients. Meropenem has a lower reported risk of seizures (0.05% to 0.8%) than does imipenem/cilastatin (2% to 7%).[43]

Another retrospective review of neurosurgery patients with gram-negative bacillary meningitis assessed treatment regimens. Briggs et al initiated therapy with ceftriaxone plus amikacin.[66] After susceptibility results, approximately half the patients remained on the initial antibiotics and the rest were changed to an alternate regimen, usually a carbapenem. These antibiotic regimens resulted in a cure of 85% of the patients.

An expert panel from The Infectious Diseases Society of America, the Surgical Infection Society, the American Society for Microbiology, and the Society of Infectious Disease Pharmacists, developed Guidelines for the Selection of Anti-infective Agents for Complicated Intra-Abdominal Infections. In choosing effective therapy, Solomkin et al found that health-care-associated intra-abdominal infections are most often acquired as complications of surgery and are caused by organisms common to the surgical site and to the specific unit or facility.[67] Intra-abdominal infections acquired in the community are caused by flora normally found at the site of perforation (stomach, intestines, or appendix).

Community-acquired intra-abdominal infections may vary from mild to severe and require treatment options as outlined in Table 6-6.[66] Nosocomial intra-abdominal infections are caused by more resistant organisms

Table 6-6: Treatment of Community-Acquired Intra-Abdominal Infections*

Infections of mild to moderate severity

- Ampicillin/sulbactam
- Cefazolin or cefuroxime plus metronidazole
- Ticarcillin/clavulanate
- Ertapenem
- Quinolones plus metronidazole

More severe infections or immunosuppressed patients

- Meropenem
- Imipenem/cilastatin
- Third- or fourth-generation cephalosporins plus metronidazole
- Ciprofloxacin plus metronidazole
- Piperacillin/tazobactam

* Definitive treatment should be based on susceptibility results.
Adapted from Solomkin[67]

and require multidrug regimens for a broader spectrum of coverage.

Narrow-spectrum antibiotic therapy is generally appropriate for patients who acquire pneumonia in the first four days of hospitalization, have no severe underlying illness, and have no prior exposure to antibiotics.

The SENTRY Antimicrobial Surveillance Program reported on antibacterial activity of 41 antimicrobials tested against more than 2,773 bacterial isolates from hospital patients with pneumonia.[46] Among US isolates of *Enterobacter* species, 90% were susceptible to cefepime, imipenem, meropenem, aminoglycosides, and fluoroquinolones.

Chapman and Perry reviewed cefepime use for hospitalized patients with pneumonia.[68] They reported that randomized clinical trials of patients with moderate to severe community-acquired or nosocomial pneumonia showed that cefepime monotherapy exhibited good clinical and bacteriological effect, including against *Enterobacter*.

Another study by Mimoz et al tested a combination of cefepime plus amikacin (Amikin®) in vitro and in vivo against a ceftazidime-resistant strain of *E cloacae* and found a synergistic response that was greater than that of either agent alone.[69] Lynch, however, questioned the benefit of adjunctive aminoglycosides because of their poor penetration into bronchopulmonary secretions and the lung, inactivation when pH is low, and potential for serious side effects, especially nephrotoxicity.[47]

Kollef recommended the use of carbapenems for empiric antimicrobial therapy,[45] although meropenem monotherapy was effective as empiric therapy in an open-label, nonrandomized trial of patients with hospital-acquired pneumonia.[70]

Treatment of empyema should begin with drainage of the infected site and treatment with clindamycin (Cleocin®) plus a third-generation cephalosporin. Suggested alternative treatment includes cefoxitin (Mefoxin®), imipenem, ticarcillin/clavulanate, piperacillin/tazobactam, or ampicillin/sulbactam.

Skin and Soft Tissue Infections

Gram-positive organisms are the most common pathogens in burn wound infections, followed later by gram-negative organisms. Early excision of the burn site is important to reduce bacterial colonization and subsequent risk of infection. Silver sulfadiazine (Silvadene®, Thermazene®) cream, silver nitrate solution, or mafenide acetate (Sulfamylon®) cream should be applied twice a day. If the wound results in sepsis, IV vancomycin plus amikacin and piperacillin (Pipracil®) is suggested, with half the daily dose of piperacillin given into subeschar tissues.

The suggested treatment for *Enterobacter* wound infections of mild to moderate severity is double-strength TMP/SMX, or amoxicillin/clavulanate. For septic wounds accompanied by fever and hospitalization, ampicillin/sulbactam, ticarcillin/clavulanate, piperacillin/tazobactam, imipenem, meropenem, or ertapenem (Invanz®) are primary options. Abscesses should be drained.

Surgical debridement of early, mild cellulitis in a patient with diabetes mellitus is important to rule out necrotizing fasciitis. For serious skin and skin structure infections, a carbapenem such as meropenem or imipenem or a β-lactam/β-lactamase inhibitor combination such as piperacillin/tazobactam should be used.

Urinary Tract Infections

Enterobacter account for 4% of all urinary isolates in the SENTRY Antimicrobial Surveillance Program.[71] Urinary tract infections continue to be a worldwide problem, especially in hospitalized patients. Treatment for acute, uncomplicated urinary tract infections, such as cystitis and urethritis, includes double-strength TMP/SMX, and if the patient is allergic to sulfa, nitrofurantoin (Macrobid®) or fosfomycin (Monurol®) can be given. Alternatives include ciprofloxacin, gatifloxacin (Tequin®), or levofloxacin (Levaquin®). Two other fluoroquinolones, moxifloxacin (Avelox®) and gemifloxacin (Factive®), however, should not be used, because neither achieves adequate concentration in urine, nor are they FDA approved for urinary tract infections.

A fluoroquinolone can be used to treat *Enterobacter* pyelonephritis. Hospitalized patients with pyelonephritis can be treated with a fluoroquinolone, ampicillin plus gentamicin, a third-generation cephalosporin, or piperacillin. Alternative therapy includes ticarcillin/clavulanate, ampicillin/sulbactam, piperacillin/tazobactam, or a carbapenem.

For complicated urinary tract infections and catheter-related urinary tract infections, a combination of ampicillin plus gentamicin, piperacillin/tazobactam, ticarcillin/clavulanate, imipenem, or meropenem are indicated with IV ciprofloxacin, gatifloxacin, or levofloxacin as alternatives. If the organism is susceptible, the patient should be switched to an oral fluoroquinolone or TMP/SMX when clinically stable and able to tolerate oral medications.

Postoperative endophthalmitis requires an immediate ophthalmology consult. Treatment consists of needle aspiration of vitreous and aqueous humor for culture before therapy. Administration of antimicrobials is done intravitreally with vancomycin and ceftazidime.

References

1.   Fok TF, Lee CH, Wong EM, et al: Risk factors for *Enterobacter* septicemia in a neonatal unit: case-control study. *Clin Infect Dis* 1998;27:1204-1209.

2.   National Nosocomial Infections Surveillance (NNIS) System report, data summary from January 1990 to May 1999, issued June 1999. *Am J Infect Control* 1999;27:520-532.

3.   Wisplinghoff H, Bischoff T, Tallent SM, et al: Nosocomial bloodstream infections in US hospitals: analysis of 24,179 cases from a prospective nationwide surveillance study. *Clin Infect Dis* 2004;39:309-317.

4.   Kang CI, Kim SH, Park WB, et al: Bloodstream infections caused by antibiotic-resistant gram-negative bacilli: risk factors for mortality and impact of inappropriate initial antimicrobial therapy on outcome. *Antimicrob Agents Chemother* 2005;49:760-766.

5.   Sanders WE Jr, Sanders CC: *Enterobacter* spp: pathogens poised to flourish at the turn of the century. *Clin Microbiol Rev* 1997;10-220-241.

6.   Chow JW, Fine MJ, Shlaes DM, et al: *Enterobacter* bacteremia: clinical features and emergence of antibiotic resistance during therapy. *Ann Intern Med* 1991;115:585-590.

7.   Russo TA: Diseases caused by gram-negative enteric bacilli. In: Braunwald E, Fauci AS, Kasper DL, et al, eds. *Harrison's Prin-*

ciples of Internal Medicine, 15th ed. New York, NY, McGraw-Hill, 2001 pp 953-960.

8.   Lehner A, Stephan R: Microbiological, epidemiological, and food safety aspects of *Enterobacter sakazakii*. *J Food Prot* 2004;67:2850-2857.

9.   Karlowsky JA, Jones ME, Thornsberry C, et al: Trends in antimicrobial susceptibilities among Enterobacteriaceae isolated from hospitalized patients in the United States from 1998 to 2001. *Antimicrob Agents Chemother* 2003;47:1672-1680.

10.   Kaye KS, Cosgrove S, Harris A, et al: Risk factors for emergence of resistance to broad-spectrum cephalosporins among *Enterobacter* spp. *Antimicrob Agents Chemother* 2001;45:2628-2630.

11.   Muller A, Lopez-Lozano JM, Bertrand X, et al: Relationship between ceftriaxone use and resistance to third-generation cephalosporins among strains of *Enterobacter cloacae*. *J Antimicrob Chemother* 2004;54:173-177.

12.   Pitout JD, Moland ES, Sanders CC, et al: Beta-lactamases and detection of β-lactam resistance in *Enterobacter* spp. *Antimicrob Agents Chemother* 1997;41:35-39.

13.   Kang CI, Kim SH, Park WB, et al: Clinical epidemiology of ciprofloxacin resistance and its relationship to broad-spectrum cephalosporin resistance in bloodstream infections caused by *Enterobacter* species. *Infect Control Hosp Epidemiol* 2005;26:88-92.

14.   Lautenbach E, Strom BL, Nachamkin I, et al: Longitudinal trends in fluoroquinolone resistance among Enterobacteriaceae isolates from inpatients and outpatients, 1989-2000: differences in the emergence and epidemiology of resistance across organisms. *Clin Infect Dis* 2004;38:655-662.

15.   Nordmann P, Mariotte S, Naas T, et al: Biochemical properties of a carbapenem-hydrolyzing beta-lactamase from *Enterobacter cloacae* and cloning of the gene into *Escherichia coli*. *Antimicrob Agents Chemother* 1993;37:939-946.

16.   Lovering AM, Bywater MJ, Holt HA, et al: Resistance of bacterial pathogens to four aminoglycosides and six other antibacterials and prevalence of aminoglycoside modifying enzymes, in 20 UK centres. *J Antimicrob Chemother* 1988;22:823-839.

17.   Maes P, Vanhoof R: A 56-month prospective surveillance study on the epidemiology of aminoglycoside resistance in a Belgian general hospital. *Scand J Infect Dis* 1992;24:495-501.

18.   Larson LL, Ramphal R: Extended-spectrum beta-lactamases. *Semin Respir Infect* 2002;17:189-194.

19.   Bell JM, Turnidge JD, Jones RN, SENTRY Asia-Pacific participants: Prevalence of extended-spectrum β-lactamase-producing *Enterobacter cloacae* in the Asia-Pacific region: results from the SENTRY Antimicrobial Surveillance Program, 1998 to 2001. *Antimicrob Agents Chemother* 2003;47:3989-3993.

20.   Charrel RN, Pages JM, De Micco P, et al: Prevalence of outer membrane porin alteration in beta–lactam antibiotic resistant *Enterobacter aerogenes*. *Antimicrob Agents Chemother* 1996;40:2854-2858.

21.   Piagnerelli M, Carlier E, Deplano A, et al: Risk factors for infection and molecular typing in patients in the intensive care unit colonized with nosocomial *Enterobacter aerogenes*. *Infect Control Hosp Epidemiol* 2002;23:452-456.

22.   Livrelli V, De Champs C, Di Martino P, et al: Adhesive properties and antibiotic resistance of *Klebsiella*, *Enterobacter*, and *Serratia* clinical isolates involved in nosocomial infections. *J Clin Microbiol* 1996;34:1963-1969.

23.   Kjolen H, Andersen BM: Handwashing and disinfection of heavily contaminated hands—effective or ineffective? *J Hosp Infect* 1992;21:61-71.

24.   Breeuwer P, Lardeau A, Peterz M, et al: Desiccation and heat tolerance of *Enterobacter sakazakii*. *J Appl Microbiol* 2003;95:967-973.

25.   Iversen C, Lane M, Forsythe SJ: The growth profile, thermotolerance and biofilm formation of *Enterobacter sakazakii* grown in infant formula milk. *Lett Appl Microbiol* 2004;38:378-382.

26.   Ferguson R, Feeney C, Chirurgi V: *Enterobacter agglomerans*-associated cotton fever. *Arch Intern Med* 1993;153:2381-2382.

27.   Stenhouse MA: *Enterobacter agglomerans* as a contaminant of blood. *Transfusion* 1992;32:86.

28.   Centers for Disease Control and Prevention: Outbreaks of gram-negative bacterial bloodstream infections traced to probable contamination of hemodialysis machines—Canada, 1995, United States, 1997; and Israel, 1997. *MMWR Morb Mortal Wkly Rep* 1998;47:55-58.

29.   Kuboyama RH, de Oliveira HB, Moretti-Branchini ML: Molecular epidemiology of systemic infection caused by *Enterobac-*

ter cloacae in a high-risk neonatal intensive care unit. *Infect Control Hosp Epidemiol* 2003;24:490-494.

30. Crowley B, Ratcliffe G: Extended-spectrum beta-lactamases in *Enterobacter cloacae*: underestimated but clinically significant! *J Antimicrob Chemother* 2003;51:1316-1317.

31. Eisenstein BI, Zaleznik DF: Enterobacteriaceae. In: Mandell GL, Bennett JE, Dolin R, eds. *Principles and Practice of Infectious Diseases*, 5th ed. Philadelphia, PA, Churchill Livingstone, 2000, pp 2294-2310.

32. Diekema DJ, Pfaller MA, Jones RN, et al: Survey of bloodstream infections due to gram-negative bacilli: frequency of occurrence and antimicrobial susceptibility of isolates collected in the United States, Canada, and Latin America for the SENTRY Antimicrobial Surveillance Program, 1997. *Clin Infect Dis* 1999;29:595-607.

33. National Nosocomial Infections Surveillance (NNIS) System: National Nosocomial Infections Surveillance (NNIS) System Report, data summary from January 1992 through June 2004, issued October 2004. *Am J Infect Control* 2004;32:470-485.

34. Cosgrove SE, Kaye KS, Eliopoulos GM, et al: Health and economic outcomes of the emergence of third-generation cephalosporin resistance in *Enterobacter* species. *Arch Intern Med* 2002;162:185-190.

35. Blot SI, Vandewoude KH, Colardyn FA: Evaluation of outcome in critically ill patients with nosocomial *Enterobacter* bacteremia: results of a matched cohort study. *Chest* 2003;123:1208-1213.

36. Calil R, Marba ST, von Nowakonski A, et al: Reduction in colonization and nosocomial infection by multiresistant bacteria in a neonatal unit after institution of educational measures and restriction in the use of cephalosporins. *Am J Infect Control* 2001;29:133-138.

37. Rochon-Edouard S, Pons JL, Veber B, et al: Comparative in vitro and in vivo study of nine alcohol-based handrubs. *Am J Infect Control* 2004;32:200-204.

38. Gordon KA, Jones RN; SENTRY participant groups (Europe, Latin America, North America): Susceptibility patterns of orally administered antimicrobials among urinary tract infection pathogens from hospitalized patients in North America; comparison report to Europe and Latin America. Results from the SENTRY an-

timicrobial surveillance program (2000). *Diagn Microbiol Infect Dis* 2003;45:295-301.

39. Stoll BJ, Hansen N, Fanaroff AA, et al: *Enterobacter sakazakii* is a rare cause of neonatal septicemia or meningitis in VLBW infants. *J Pediatr* 2004;144:821-823.

40. Tunkel AR, Fisch MJ, Schlein A, et al: *Enterobacter endocarditis. Scand J Infect Dis* 1992;24:233-240.

41. Wolff MA, Young CL, Ramphal R: Antibiotic therapy for *Enterobacter meningitis*: a retrospective review of 13 episodes and review of the literature. *Clin Infect Dis* 1993;16:772-777.

42. Willis J, Robinson JE: *Enterobacter sakazakii* meningitis in neonates. *Pediatr Infect Dis J* 1988;7:196-199.

43. Parodi S, Lechner A, Osih R, et al: Nosocomial *Enterobacter meningitis*: risk factors, management, and treatment outcomes. *Clin Infect Dis* 2003;37:159-166.

44. Finegold SM, Johnson CC: Lower respiratory tract infection. *Am J Med* 1985;79:73-77.

45. Kollef MH: Appropriate empiric antimicrobial therapy of nosocomial pneumonia: the role of the carbapenems. *Respir Care* 2004;49:1530-1541.

46. Mathai D, Lewis MT, Kugler KC, et al: Antibacterial activity of 41 antimicrobials tested against over 2773 bacterial isolates from hospitalized patients with pneumonia: I-results from the SENTRY Antimicrobial Surveillance Program (North America, 1998). *Diagn Microbiol Infect Dis* 2001;39:105-116.

47. Sanchez-Nieto JM, Torres A, Garcia-Cordoba F, et al: Impact of invasive and noninvasive quantitative culture sampling on outcome of ventilator-associated pneumonia: a pilot study. *Am J Respir Crit Care Med* 1998;157:371-376.

48. Lynch JP III: Hospital-acquired pneumonia. Risk factors, microbiology, and treatment. *Chest* 2001;119(2 suppl):373S-384S.

49. Deusch E, End A, Grimm M, et al: Early bacterial infections in lung transplant recipients. *Chest* 1993;104:1412-1416.

50. Ganelin RS, Ellis M: Cellulitis caused by *Enterobacter cloacae. J Infect* 1992;24:218-219.

51. Palmer DL, Kuritsky JN, Lapham SC, et al: *Enterobacter mediastinitis* following cardiac surgery. *Infect Control* 1985;6:115-119.

52. Jarvis WR, Martone WJ: Predominant pathogens in hospital infections. *J Antimicrob Chemother* 1992;29(suppl A):19-24.

53. Mirza GE, Karakucuk S, Doganay M, et al: Postoperative endophthalmitis caused by an *Enterobacter* species. *J Hosp Infect* 1994;26:167-172.

54. Bouza E, Cercenado E: *Klebsiella* and *Enterobacter*: antibiotic resistance and treatment implications. *Semin Respir Infect* 2002;17:215-230.

55. Bradford PA: Extended-spectrum beta-lactamases in the 21st century: characterization, epidemiology, and detection of this important resistance threat. *Clin Microbio Rev* 2001;14:933-951.

56. Levison ME, Mailapur YV, Pradhan SE, et al: Regional occurrence of plasmid-mediated SHV-7, an extended-spectrum beta-lactamase, in *Enterobacter cloacae* in Philadelphia teaching hospitals. *Clin Infect Dis* 2002;35:1551-1554.

57. Jacobs RA, Guglielmo BJ: Anti-infective chemotherapeutic & antibiotic agents. In: Tierney LM Jr, McPhee SJ, Papadakis MA, eds. *Current Medical Diagnosis and Treatment*, 43rd ed. New York, NY, Lange Medical Books/McGraw-Hill, 2004 pp 1486-1526.

58. Setia U, Gross PA: Bacteremia in a community hospital: spectrum and mortality. *Arch Intern Med* 1977;137:1698-1701.

59. Weinstein MP, Murphy JR, Reller LB, et al: The clinical significance of positive blood cultures: a comprehensive analysis of 500 episodes of bacteremia and fungemia in adults. II. Clinical observations, with special reference to factors influencing prognosis. *Rev Infect Dis* 1983;5:54-70.

60. Chambers HF: Infectious diseases: bacterial & chlamydial. In: Tierney LM Jr, McPhee SJ, Papadakis MA, eds. *Current Medical Diagnosis and Treatment*. 43rd ed. New York, NY, Lange Medical Books/McGraw-Hill; 2004:1337-1379.

61. Pfaller MA, Jones RN, Doern GV, et al: Bacterial pathogens isolated from patients with bloodstream infection: frequencies of occurrence and antimicrobial susceptibility patterns from the SENTRY Antimicrobial Surveillance Program (United States and Canada, 1997). *Antimicrob Agents Chemother* 1998;42:1762-1770.

62. Pai H, Hong JY, Byeon JH, et al: High prevalence of extended-spectrum blactamase-producing strains among blood isolates of

Enterobacter spp. collected in a tertiary hospital during an 8-year period and their antimicrobial susceptibility patterns. *Antimicrob Agents Chemother* 2004;48:3159-3161.

63. Critchley IA, Sahm DF, Kelly LJ, et al: In vitro synergy studies using aztreonam and fluoroquinolone combinations against six species of gram-negative bacilli. *Chemotherapy* 2003;49:44-48.

64. Liu CP, Wang NY, Lee CM, et al: Nosocomial and community-acquired *Enterobacter cloacae* bloodstream infection: risk factors for and prevalence of SHV-12 in multiresistant isolates in a medical centre. *J Hosp Infect* 2004;58:63-77.

65. Jung R, Husain M, Choi MK, et al: Synergistic activities of moxifloxacin combined with piperacillin-tazobactam or cefepime against *Klebsiella pneumoniae*, *Enterobacter cloacae*, and *Acinetobacter baumannii* clinical isolates. *Antimicrob Agents Chemother* 2004;48:1055-1057.

66. Briggs S, Ellis-Pegler R, Raymond N, et al: Gram-negative bacillary meningitis after cranial surgery or trauma in adults. *Scand J Infect Dis* 2004;36:165-173.

67. Solomkin JS, Mazuski JE, Baron EJ, et al: Guidelines for the selection of anti-infective agents for complicated intra-abdominal infections. *Clin Infect Dis* 2003;37:997-1005.

68. Chapman TM, Perry CM: Cefepime: a review of its use in the management of hospitalized patients with pneumonia. *Am J Respir Med* 2003;2:75-107.

69. Mimoz O, Jacolot A, Padoin C, et al: Cefepime and amikacin synergy in vitro and in vivo against a ceftazidime-resistant strain of *Enterobacter cloacae*. *J Antimicrob Chemother* 1998;41:367-372.

70. Berman SJ, Fogarty CM, Fabian T, et al: Meropenem monotherapy for the treatment of hospital-acquired pneumonia: results of a multicenter trial. *J Chemother* 2004;16:362-371.

71. Gordon KA, Jones RN, SENTRY participant groups (Europe, Latin America, North America): Susceptibility patterns of orally administered antimicrobials among urinary tract infection pathogens from hospitalized patients in North America: comparison report to Europe and Latin America. Results from the SENTRY Antimicrobial Surveillance Program (2000). *Diagn Microbiol Infect Dis* 2003;45:295-301.

Chapter 7

Pseudomonas aeruginosa

The emergence of serious infections caused by multidrug-resistant organisms poses a major threat, especially to intensive care unit (ICU) patients. *Pseudomonas aeruginosa* is a particular threat because it causes a wide range of acute and chronic infections and is one of the most difficult pathogens to treat.[1-3] *P aeruginosa* exhibits intrinsic resistance to multiple classes of antimicrobials and can acquire resistance during treatment.[4,5] In addition, acquired resistance is rapidly increasing among *P aeruginosa* strains, especially in ICUs and in patients with cystic fibrosis.[3]

Clinical Microbiology

P aeruginosa is an aerobic, nonfermentative, gram-negative rod. It is a small, motile bacillus with a single flagellum at one end. Many *P aeruginosa* organisms produce pyocyanin, a blue-green pigment that plays a role in virulence.[3,6] *Pseudomonas* can be found in soil, water, vegetation, and animals. It grows almost anywhere, but especially thrives in moist environments. *P aeruginosa* seldom causes community-acquired infections in healthy individuals, but is a leading nosocomial pathogen.[1,3,7]

Mechanisms of Resistance

Strains of *P aeruginosa* exhibit multiple intrinsic- and acquired-resistance mechanisms that confer resistance to numerous antimicrobials.[4,5,8] The major mechanisms of resistance include hyperproduction of β-lactamases, reduction in outer membrane permeability, efflux pump systems, and plasmid-mediated aminoglycoside-modifying enzymes.[4,5,8] Mobile genetic elements may carry genes for multiple enzymes, conferring multidrug resistance.[9]

Efflux systems in *P aeruginosa* efficiently pump specific antimicrobial agents out of the bacterial cell, reducing their intracellular concentrations and thereby reducing susceptibility to these agents.[4] At least four multidrug efflux pumps have been identified in *P aeruginosa*, and additional pump systems are being investigated.[10]

Porins in the outer membrane of gram-negative cells function as channels for the passage of molecules into and out of the bacterial cell. The loss of the porin OprD is associated with resistance to imipenem and decreased susceptibility to meropenem.[5] Of particular concern is the combination of up-regulating efflux, loss of OprD, and impermeability to aminoglycosides, which results in resistance to every drug class except polymyxins.[5]

Pathogenicity and Virulence

P aeruginosa is an opportunistic pathogen, rarely causing disease in healthy individuals but capable of virulence when normal host defenses are breached. The risk for infection is greatly increased when surgery, trauma, burns, or indwelling devices create a break in cutaneous or mucosal barriers; when use of broad-spectrum antibiotics disrupts the protective function of the normal flora; or when immunologic defense mechanisms have been compromised (eg, from chemotherapy, cystic fibrosis, diabetes mellitus, or AIDS).[3,7]

Pathogenesis is a complex process in *P aeruginosa*. The first step begins with adherence and colonization of *P aeruginosa* to epithelial tissue. While primarily responsible for motility of the organism, the flagellum may also act as an adhesin, along with pili, which are hairlike organelles extending outward from the lipopolysaccharide layer of the cell. Alginate, a mucoid exopolysaccharide produced by most strains of *Pseudomonas*, plays a role in colonization and infection of the respiratory tract in patients with cystic fibrosis.[3,7] Alginate also comprises the matrix that surrounds mutant bacteria to form a biofilm in cystic fibrosis patients. The matrix helps protect the bacteria from phagocytosis, the action of complement, and antimicrobial agents.

Once adherence to the epithelium and colonization have been achieved, P aeruginosa produces a variety of extracellular virulence factors that cause tissue damage, bloodstream invasion, and dissemination of the pathogen (Figure 7-1). These virulence factors include exotoxins A and S, hemolysins phospholipase C and rhamnolipid, and several proteases (LasB elastase, LasA elastase, and alkaline protease).[3,7]

The exotoxins inhibit protein synthesis and the hemolysins appear to synergistically break down lipids and lecithin, as well as contribute to tissue invasion. The two elastases destroy the protein elastin, which is a part of human lung tissue responsible for lung expansion and contraction and imparts resilience to blood vessels. The elastases have been found in the sputum of cystic fibrosis patients during exacerbation of their disease.[11]

A cell-to-cell signaling system, termed quorum sensing, regulates the production and secretion of many virulence factors. This system appears to give P aeruginosa the ability to overcome host defenses by coordinating the expression of virulence genes in an entire bacterial population, once a critical density is sensed. When this point is reached, the production of extracellular virulence factors may be sufficient to breach host defenses, leading to invasion, dissemination, systemic inflammatory response syndrome, and ultimately, death.

An additional mechanism that enhances virulence is the type III secretion apparatus. This is a complex array of transmembrane proteins that facilitate injection of certain virulence factors from the bacterium directly into the host cells, bypassing immune defenses.[3,12] In vitro

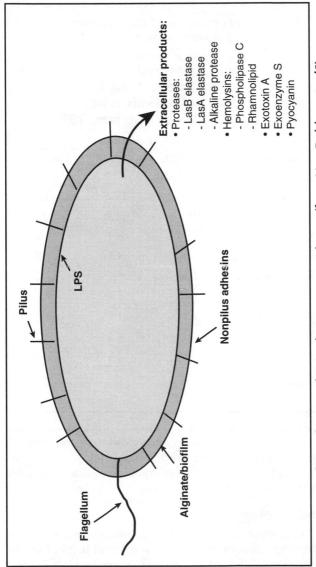

Figure 7-1: Virulence factors of *Pseudomonas aeruginosa* (from Van Delden et al[7]).

Table 7-1: Frequency of Occurrence of Bacterial Pathogens Causing Pneumonias in Hospitalized Patients in the US and Canada (SENTRY Antimicrobial Surveillance Program, 1997)

	Percentage of total		
Organisms	United States	Canada	Combined
S aureus	23.0	22.5	22.9
P aeruginosa	18.2	17.6	18.1
H influenzae	10.1	11.0	10.3
Klebsiella	8.7	8.7	8.7
S pneumoniae	7.6	8.1	7.7
Enterobacter	7.8	6.1	7.4
E coli	4.4	5.7	4.7
S maltophilia	3.5	3.7	3.6
M catarrhalis	3.0	4.2	3.3
S marcescens	2.6	2.4	2.6

From Jones[14]

studies show that *Pseudomonas* exhibiting the type III phenotype has a 6-fold greater risk of mortality in patients with lower respiratory tract infections caused by *P aeruginosa*.

Epidemiology

Pseudomonas aeruginosa is an important pathogen with multidrug-resistant strains distributed worldwide. The European Prevalence of Infection in Intensive Care (EPIC) study found that *P aeruginosa* (28.7%) was second only to *Staphylococcus aureus* (30.1%) as the most frequently isolated organism in ICUs.[13] Data from the SENTRY Antimicrobial Surveillance Program showed *P aeruginosa* to be the second leading cause of pneumonia[14] (Table 7-1) and skin and soft tissue infections in North America,[15] the third most frequent cause of bloodstream infections in North America and Latin America,[16] and the fourth most common cause of urinary tract infections in North America.[17] Data from The Surveillance Network (TSN) indicates an increasing trend to multidrug resistance among *P aeruginosa* strains[5] (Table 7-2), and the National Nosocomial Infections Surveillance (NNIS) system reported increases of 15%, 9%, and 20% *in P aeruginosa* resistance to imipenem, quinolones, and third-generation cephalosporins, respectively.[18]

Rates of carriage of *P aeruginosa* are fairly low, except among patients who have serious underlying illness, have been exposed to the hospital environment, have received prior antibiotic therapy, or are immunocompromised. Among these patients, colonization with *P aeruginosa* generally precedes infection. *Pseudomonas* infections are usually nosocomially acquired, but HIV-infected patients are also at risk for community-acquired *P aeruginosa* infections.

Many reservoirs have been identified in the hospital where *Pseudomonas* organisms can grow and from which they can be transmitted to patients via the hands of healthcare workers. Respiratory equipment, sinks and water taps, flowers, vegetables, and even cleaning solutions and disinfectants are potential reservoirs.[3] Outbreaks of *Pseudomonas* infections have been traced to use of contaminated iodophor solution,[19] to recreational and hydrotherapy pools,[20] to bronchoscopes with a loose port,[21] and to an endoscope used for diagnostic and treatment purposes of biliary disorders, even after undergoing routine high-level disinfection.[22]

Table 7-2: Trends in Resistance Among *Pseudomonas aeruginosa* Isolates in the US

Antimicrobial agent	Percentage resistance, by patient isolate	
	All	Inpatient
Ceftazidime	11.5	13.2
Piperacillin	15.8	17.9
Imipenem	14.2	15.5
Amikacin	7.1	6.1
Gentamicin	19.1	18.9
Ciprofloxacin	29.5	31.2

*cystic fibrosis

Resistance among P aeruginosa *strains*

Multidrug-resistant *P aeruginosa* represents a crisis in therapeutic management. In addition to intrinsic resistance, acquired resistance is steadily increasing, especially in ICUs and in patients with cystic fibrosis.[3] The growing use of antibiotics, increased severity of illness in hospital patients, liberal use of immunosuppressive therapies, and inadequate control measures all contribute to the rise in *Pseudomonas* strains that are resistant to multiple antimicrobials.

Additional risk factors for antibiotic-resistant infections include mechanical ventilation of at least seven days, prior use of a broad-spectrum antibiotic, prolonged hospital stay, or residence in a long-term-care facility[4] (Table 7-3).

Prior use of antibiotics is a risk factor for subsequent development of resistance. For example, studies have shown that use of quinolones results in a high risk for subsequent development of infections with quinolone-resistant organisms.[23,24] A study by Zervos and colleagues ex-

Percentage resistance, by patient isolate		
ICU	Outpatient	CF* sputum
18.2	8.3	18.8
23.5	12.0	19.8
22.5	11.4	14.2
6.0	8.8	26.4
22.3	18.7	41.1
32.2	27.0	23.3

Adapted from Livermore[5]

amined the relationship between fluoroquinolone use and the susceptibilities of 11 bacterial pathogens to fluoroquinolones in 10 US hospitals.[25] Between 1991 and 2000, *P aeruginosa* isolates showed a 25.1% decrease in fluoroquinolone susceptibility.

Poole reported on aminoglycoside resistance in *P aeruginosa* and concluded that the increasing prevalence of strains with multiple aminoglycoside-modifying enzymes and of efflux systems that export the drug threaten to compromise use of the entire class of aminoglycosides.[9]

Because *P aeruginosa* can rapidly acquire resistance to cephalosporins and fluoroquinolones, carbapenems have become an option for treatment.[26] Mutant strains of *P aeruginosa*, however, confer resistance to carbapenems through hyperproduction of β-lactamases. Importantly, these strains are able to accept transferable β-lactamase genes that confer carbapenem resistance at a level that results in clinical failure.[26]

Table 7-3: Factors Associated With *Pseudomonas aeruginosa* Infections

- Disruption of cutaneous of mucosal barriers
  - burn injury
  - dermatitis
  - penetrating trauma
  - surgery
  - endotracheal intubation
  - indwelling central venous catheters
  - urinary catheterization
  - injection drug use
- Disruption of normal bacterial flora
  - broad-spectrum antibiotic therapy
  - exposure to the hospital environment
- Immunosuppression
- Neutropenia
- Qualitative white blood cell defects
- Hypogammaglobulinemia
- Defective cell-mediated immunity
- Extremes of age
- Diabetes mellitus
- Steroid therapy
- Cystic fibrosis
- Cancer
- AIDS

Adapted from Ohl[3]

The Tracking Resistance in the United States Today (TRUST) surveillance study reported on antimicrobial susceptibility rates for clinical isolates, including *P aeruginosa,* from 2001 to 2003.[27] Data showed that while resistance rates for ciprofloxacin, levofloxacin, ceftazidime, and gentamicin remained relatively stable, resistance to imipenem nearly doubled, from 8.8% in 2001 to 16.0% in 2003.

Costs and Prevention

Infection with *P aeruginosa* is costly, both in economic impact and in the health of patients infected. The attributable mortality for *P aeruginosa* bacteremia is 34%[28] and even higher in AIDS patients infected with this organism.[29] The organism is also responsible for pneumonia and septicemia among immunocompromised patients, with attributable deaths approaching 30%.[30]

Carmeli and coworkers examined the clinical and economic effects of antibiotic resistance in patients hospitalized with *P aeruginosa.*[31] Emergence of resistance was found to significantly increase length of hospital stay as well as total cost.

In addition to strict hand washing or use of antiseptics and appropriate use of gloves, suggested interventions to help reduce incidence of *Pseudomonas* infections include early appropriate antimicrobial therapy, rotating empiric antibiotic regimens, restricting use of third-generation cephalosporins, and administration of antimicrobials for the shortest effective duration.[32,33]

Clinical Infections

Pseudomonas causes a broad range of infections, including respiratory tract and urinary tract infections, bacteremia, endocarditis, and infections of the central nervous system, ear, eye, bones and joints, skin and soft tissues. Primarily an opportunistic nosocomial pathogen, *P aeruginosa* is the second most common cause of infections in ICUs and a frequent cause of ventilator-associated pneumonia (VAP).[34]

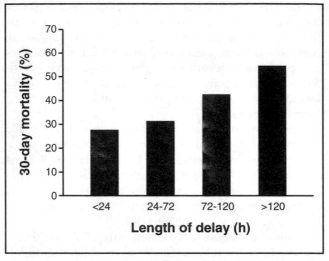

Figure 7-2: Thirty-day mortality rates according to the length of delay in receiving antimicrobial therapy. Note: The delay of >120 h includes patients who received ineffective definitive antimicrobial therapy. (Adapted from Kang[35]).

Bloodstream Infections

Bacteremia. *Pseudomonas* is an important cause of life-threatening bloodstream infections in immunocompromised patients (especially neutropenia) and often occurs along with other comorbid conditions. Primary bacteremia has no identifiable source of infection and secondary bacteremia arises from a known focus of infection.

Studies by Kang and coworkers and Osmon and colleagues verified that delay in receiving appropriate antibiotic therapy is the most important predictor of mortality in patients with *P aeruginosa* bacteremia.[35,36] And, as the length of the delay increases, so does the risk of death (Figure 7-2). Kang and Osmon also compared *S aureus* bacteremia to *P aeruginosa* bacteremia and reported that although *S aureus* bacteremia is more common than bacteremia caused by *P aeruginosa*, bloodstream infections from *P aeruginosa* are more likely to be associated with lack of clinical response to initial therapy and with greater risk of mortality. Kang cited inappropriate antimicrobial therapy, septic shock, pneumonia, and severe underlying disease as independent risk factors for development of *P aeruginosa* bacteremia.

Endocarditis. *P aeruginosa* infects native heart valves primarily in injection drug users, resulting in right-sided endocarditis. When *Pseudomonas* infects prosthetic heart valves, left-sided endocarditis ensues. Right-sided *P aeruginosa* endocarditis is usually subacute and may be associated with septic pulmonary emboli. Left-sided infection is more likely to be acute and may present as intractable heart failure or large systemic emboli. Multiple valve infections are common with *P aeruginosa*.[3]

Intra-abdominal infections. *P aeruginosa* infection at a surgical site and bacteremic seeding can result in intra-abdominal infections. Patients on peritoneal dialysis may also acquire *P aeruginosa* peritonitis from infections of the peritoneal catheter.

Kumar and colleagues described an unusual mode of transmission in a study of a *Pseudomonas* outbreak in organ transplant recipients.[37] *P aeruginosa* was transmitted from a donor innominate artery graft to several recipients. The donor was not bacteremic but had tracheal colonization of *P aeruginosa* that likely contaminated the artery. Infections at vascular anastomosis sites with graft loss occurred in three patients (liver, kidney, and kidney-pancreas), and severe pneumonia developed in the lung patient.

Respiratory Tract Infections

Pneumonia. Neutropenic and mechanically ventilated patients are at greatest risk of *P aeruginosa* pneumonia. In these patients, mortality exceeds 30%.[1] Colonization of the upper respiratory tract is the major mechanism responsible for nosocomial pneumonia.

Community-acquired pneumonia caused by *P aeruginosa* is uncommon and occurs mostly in patients with underlying disease, including cystic fibrosis, cancer, aplastic anemia, chronic obstructive pulmonary disease, AIDS, and bronchiectasis.[1] It has, however, been known to occur in previously healthy persons and can rapidly progress.

Ventilator-associated pneumonia (VAP) can be classified as early onset, which develops in the first 4 days of mechanical ventilation, or late onset, which develops 5 or more days after initiation of mechanical ventilation. Early onset VAP tends to be less severe and has a better prognosis than does late onset VAP. *P aeruginosa* is almost always associated with late-onset VAP, with multidrug resistance adding to the increased mortality of VAP.

The endotracheal tube used in mechanically ventilated patients is a significant factor in VAP infections. Bacteria readily colonize the tube, forming a biofilm that is resistant to antibiotics. In a study by Berra and coworkers, endotracheal tubes coated with antiseptics inhibited biofilm formation, resulting in a reduction in tracheal colonization and prevention of lung bacterial colonization.[38]

Cystic fibrosis. *P aeruginosa* plays an important role in the pathogenesis of cystic fibrosis. In early childhood, respiratory infections in cystic fibrosis patients are commonly caused by *S aureus* and *Haemophilus influenzae*, but later, *P aeruginosa* is the primary bacterial pathogen.[1] Chronic colonization with *Pseudomonas* leads to progressive decline in respiratory function and increased morbidity and mortality. Some 70% to 80% of cystic fibrosis patients become colonized with *P aeruginosa*.[39] Mucoid-producing strains of *P aeruginosa* contribute to the tenacity of the organism, as does its propensity to form biofilm.

AIDS patients. Patients with advanced stages of AIDS are particularly at risk for *P aeruginosa* infections, especially pneumonia. Unlike most *Pseudomonas* infections in non-AIDS patients, which are hospital acquired, most *P aeruginosa* infections in this population are community-acquired.[3] Relapsing bronchopulmonary infection is often chronic and bacteremia is often recurrent in AIDS patients with *P aeruginosa* pneumonia.

Skin and soft tissue infections. Breaks in the skin from trauma, burn injury, skin ulceration, or dermatitis can provide a portal for *P aeruginosa* and result in pyoderma, especially under moist conditions. Extensive third-degree burns are at risk for *Pseudomonas* wound sepsis and are associated with an extremely high mortality rate.[3]

Abscesses, cellulitis, vesicular and pustular lesions, and bullae are also clinical manifestations of *P aeruginosa* infection. Diffuse maculopapular and vesiculopustular rashes are associated with exposure to hot tubs, spas, physiotherapy pools, and swimming pools that are contaminated with *Pseudomonas*. Diabetic patients are particularly at risk for Fournier's gangrene, a potentially life-threatening infection from *P aeruginosa*.

Urinary tract infections. *Pseudomonas* is a common pathogen in urinary tract infections (UTIs).[3] Infection may result after instrumentation, urinary catheterization, surgery, or obstruction. Prostate infection and urinary calculi may be sources for chronic or recurrent infection. UTIs caused by *Pseudomonas* are often chronic, resistant to antimicrobial therapy, and recurrent. Patients with indwelling urinary catheters, paraplegia, or alteration in urinary tract anatomy after diversion procedures commonly have chronic *P aeruginosa* UTIs.[3]

Additional P aeruginosa *infections*

Ear infections. *P aeruginosa* is the predominant pathogen associated with external otitis and often causes inflammation or maceration, including 'swimmer's ear' under moist conditions. Malignant external otitis is a progressively destructive invasion of the soft tissue, cartilage, and cortical bone when *P aeruginosa* penetrates the external auditory canal. It occurs predominantly in elderly diabetic patients and can progress to osteomyelitis at the base of the skull, nerve damage, and loss of hearing.[3]

Eye infections. *P aeruginosa* causes endophthalmitis and bacterial keratitis or corneal ulcers. Corneal abrasions or trauma provide entry for the organism. Contaminated contact lens solutions can be a source of infection. Corneal ulcers may occur following eye surgery, in burn or coma patients, and in ICU patients. Endophthalmitis caused by *Pseudomonas* requires immediate treatment because it progresses rapidly and can threaten sight.

Bone and joint infections. Complicated UTIs, genitourinary instrumentation or surgery, and injection drug use may lead to vertebral osteomyelitis caused by *P aeruginosa*. Puncture wounds, compound fractures, sternotomy, and spread from sites of cellulitis and ischemic ulceration are portals of entry for *P aeruginosa* into bones and joints.

Central nervous system infections. Head trauma, surgery, or diagnostic procedures can result in *Pseudomonas* infection, which may extend into the central nervous system (CNS) and brain, causing meningitis or brain abscesses. Bacteremic spread from a distant focus of infection is also possible. Primary CNS infections with *P aeruginosa* generally occur only in immunocompromised patients.

Treatment

Because *P aeruginosa* has shown resistance to multiple antimicrobials, initial antibiotic selection should consider local patterns of antimicrobial susceptibility. Definitive treatment should be based on results of susceptibility tests of isolates from the infection (Table 7-4). In general, acute infections should be treated aggressively for the shortest effective duration. But chronic infections involving extensive tissue injury, prosthetic or foreign material, alteration in normal anatomy, or poor response to antibiotics may require treatment for extended periods.[3]

Table 7-4: Antimicrobials Active Against *Pseudomonas aeruginosa*

Antipseudomonal penicillins
- Piperacillin
- Piperacillin/ tazobactam
- Mezlocillin
- Ticarcillin
- Ticarcillin/ clavulanate

Antipseudomonal cephalosporins
- Ceftazidime*
- Cefepime

Carbapenems*
- Imipenem/cilastatin
- Meropenem

Monobactams
- Aztreonam

Aminoglycosides*
- Tobramycin
- Gentamicin
- Amikacin

Fluoroquinolones*
- Ciprofloxacin
- Levofloxacin

*Some strains may develop resistance to these agents during therapy.
Adapted from Ohl[3]

Pharmacokinetic/pharmacodynamic Modeling

Studies have shown that pharmacokinetic (PK) and pharmacodynamic (PD) parameters play an important role in the management of *P aeruginosa* infections.[40,41] Three pharmacodynamic parameters related to the minimum inhibitory concentration (MIC) of an antimicrobial agent are likely to be related to response to the agent: the area under the concentration time curve (AUC) during a 24-hour dosing interval relative to the MIC of the organism (AUC_{0-24}/MIC), the maximum serum concentration of the antibiotic relative to the MIC (C_{max}/MIC), and the percentage of a dosing interval in which the serum concentration is above the MIC (%T>MIC).[40]

Critically ill patients have altered PKs that affect metabolism, distribution, and clearance of antimicrobials. Maintaining the serum concentration of an antimicrobial agent at optimal serum concentration is more accurately determined using PK/PD models than by simply relying on in vitro susceptibilities and MIC breakpoints.

Combination Therapy

Combination therapy with two antipseudomonal antimicrobials is the preferred method of treatment of *P aeruginosa*, especially for severe or life-threatening infections and especially in the immunocompromised host.[1-3,34,42] While some studies show no difference between monotherapy with an effective agent and combination therapy, other studies show a reduction in the emergence of *Pseudomonas* resistance during treatment with combination therapy.[1] The wisdom behind combination therapy is supported by in vitro studies. Suggested benefits to combination therapy are threefold: to increase efficacy, to achieve additive or synergistic killing, and to prevent emergence of antimicrobial resistance. Initial combination therapy that provides broad coverage may improve the chance of providing effective empirical coverage, which is an important factor in reducing mortality in severe *P aeruginosa* infections.[4]

Bloodstream Infections

Bacteremia. When the source of *P aeruginosa* bacteremia is a central venous catheter, removal of the catheter is essential to prevent relapse in treatment.[43] Once the catheter is removed, monotherapy may be effective, based on susceptibility tests.[3] Data from the SENTRY Antimicrobial Surveillance Program indicated that meropenem (Merrem®), imipenem/cilastatin (Primaxin®), and cefepime (Maxipime®) were the most active antimicrobials tested against all gram-negative isolates.[16]

Combination therapy, at least as empirical therapy until results of susceptibility tests are completed, has become an important approach to treatment of *P aeruginosa* bacteremia.[44,45] A meta-analysis by Safdar and colleagues studied the benefits of combination therapy in reducing mortality in gram-negative bacteremia. They found a reduction in mortality of approximately 50% when combination therapy was used *for P aeruginosa* bacteremia.

In vitro synergy has been demonstrated against *P aeruginosa* with an antipseudomonal penicillin plus an aminoglycoside.[3,44] Alternative treatment consists of an antipseudomonal penicillin plus intravenous (IV) ciprofloxacin (Cipro®) or a combination of an antipseudomonal cephalosporin, aztreonam (Azactam®), or carbapenem plus an aminoglycoside or IV ciprofloxacin.[3]

Mendelson and coworkers examined combination therapy for treatment of bacteremia in AIDS patients.[29] Patients treated with an antipseudomonal β-lactam or aztreonam plus an aminoglycoside had higher response rates than did patients treated with a single agent.

Endocarditis. Treatment for endocarditis follows the same guidelines as for bacteremia. Valve replacement is often necessary for endocarditis caused by *P aeruginosa*, especially in patients with resistant organisms.

Intra-abdominal infections. Intra-abdominal infections are often polymicrobial, requiring complicated treatment regimens. For *P aeruginosa* coverage, an aminoglycoside plus an antipseudomonal penicillin is the treatment of choice. Alternate options include ceftazidime (Ceptaz®, Fortaz®), imipenem, meropenem, or aztreonam, either alone or with an aminoglycoside; or ciprofloxacin, either alone or with piperacillin/tazobactam (Zosyn®), ceftazidime, or cefepime.[46] Piperacillin/tazobactam and cefepime may also be used alone if the organism is susceptibile. An investigation by Erasmo and coworkers showed piperacillin/tazobactam to be as safe and effective as imipenem/cilastatin for intra-abdominal infections from *P aeruginosa*.[47]

Respiratory Tract Infections

Pneumonia. Combination therapy is often used for severe pneumonia if *P aeruginosa* is suspected or confirmed by culture. Two frequently used combinations are an aminoglycoside plus an antipseudomonal β-lactam, or a fluoroquinolone plus an antipseudomonal β-lactam. The aminoglycoside/β-lactam combination is synergistic, while a fluoroquinolone, such as ciprofloxacin, and β-lactam combination have the advantage of better tissue and respiratory secretion penetration over an aminoglycoside, plus a less toxic safety profile.[1,42]

There is a risk, however, of increasing the development of resistance among *P aeruginosa* when a fluoroquinolone is used. As with treatment of *P aeruginosa* bacteremia or endocarditis, alternate choices include an antipseudomonal penicillin plus ciprofloxacin or a combination of an antipseudomonal cephalosporin, aztreonam, or carbapenem plus an aminoglycoside or ciprofloxacin.

Studies by Burgess and colleagues and West and coworkers found that 750 mg of levofloxacin (Levaquin®) combined with a β-lactam provides an alternative to an aminoglycoside-containing regimen.[2,48] In a 7-year study of critically ill ICU patients, Linden and associates used colistin (polymyxin E) as 'salvage therapy' in patients with panresistant *P aeruginosa* infections.[8] The most common types of infections were pneumonia and intra-abdominal infections.

Colistin resistance is rare, but because of a history of nephrotoxic and neurotoxic adverse effects, use of this older antimicrobial has been generally reserved for nonsystemic applications. However, with emerging resistance, the systemic use of this agent is increasing.

Another polymyxin, polymyxin B, was studied by Sobieszczyk et al in 25 critically ill patients.[49] Aerosolized and IV polymyxin B were found to be well tolerated with a low incidence of adverse effects. More controlled trials are needed for this agent, but it appears to have potential for use in combination therapy of multidrug-resistant *P aeruginosa* respiratory tract infections.

Cystic Fibrosis

The standard of care for acute exacerbation of cystic fibrosis (CF) respiratory infection is the administration of a β-lactam plus an aminoglycoside for 10 to 14 days.[1] An additional treatment is cyclical administration of inhaled tobramycin. Several clinical studies have confirmed that the use of a nebulized solution of tobramycin effectively reduces lower airway *P aeruginosa* density and improves pulmonary function in patients with CF.[50-52] Hodson and coworkers tested nebulized tobramycin against nebulized colistin and found that tobramycin significantly improved lung function in patients with CF, but that colistin did not.

Skin and Soft Tissue Infections

Drainage of abscesses and debridement are necessary treatments for wound infections and are especially important in burn wounds. Early excision of burned and necrotic tissue greatly decreases the mortality associated with extensive burns.[53] Application of topical antimicrobials, such as silver sulfadiazine (Silvadene®) and mafenide acetate creams (Sulfamylon Cream®) and silver nitrate help reduce the risk of bacterial colonization of the site. Mafenide has better penetration and broader activity than silver sulfadiazine.

Antibiotic therapy for *P aeruginosa* wounds is a combination of an antipseudomonal penicillin plus an aminoglycoside, with alternatives similar to those for bacteremia, endocarditis, and pneumonia. Amikacin, cefepime, and carbapenems were the most active agents in the SENTRY Antimicrobial Surveillance Program data.[15]

Urinary Tract Infections

When urinary stones or urinary catheters are the foci of *Pseudomonas* infection, they should be removed. Monotherapy with ciprofloxacin, either oral or IV, is generally the preferred therapy. Alternate options include an aminoglycoside, antipseudomonal penicillin, cephalosporin, or carbapenem.[3] The dosage should be reduced for patients with renal insufficiency.

Ear Infections

Treatment of acute otitis externa, or swimmer's ear, consists of cleansing the canal with an alcohol-acetic acid mixture and administration of topical antibiotic eardrops, such as polymyxin-neomycin, 4 times a day for 5 days.

Malignant external otitis, which primarily occurs in elderly diabetic patients, can be life-threatening as it slowly extends into adjacent soft tissue, mastoid and temporal bones, and across the base of the skull. Surgical debridement is usually necessary in addition to 4 to 6 weeks of antimicrobial therapy.

For early or limited infection, oral ciprofloxacin may be used; otherwise, an antipseudomonal cephalosporin, carbapenem, or IV ciprofloxacin are the first choices for treatment. Alternate options include an antipseudomonal penicillin or cephalosporin plus an aminoglycoside.

Eye Infections

Aminoglycoside eye drops are administered for *P aeruginosa* keratitis or corneal ulceration. A topical solution of tobramycin should be used, with or without administration of a topical solution of piperacillin or ticarcillin.[3] Ciprofloxacin (Ciloxan®) or ofloxacin (Floxin Otic™) 0.3% topical solution are alternate choices.

Endophthalmitis caused by *Pseudomonas* usually requires surgical vitrectomy. Antimicrobial therapy is the same as for keratitis and corneal ulceration, but also includes intravitreal amikacin or ceftazidime. Ozkiris and coworkers investigated the use of intravitreal piperacillin/tazobactam in the treatment of experimental *P aeruginosa* endophthalmitis in an animal model and concluded piperacillin/tazobactam may be as effective as ceftazidime.[54]

Bone and joint infections

Surgical debridement may be necessary for bone or joint infections that are chronic or associated with trauma. Treatment is similar to that of bacteremia, endocarditis, and pneumonia, with antipseudomonal penicillin plus an aminoglycoside as the treatment of choice. An antipseudomonal cephalosporin, aztreonam, fluoroquinolone, or carbapenem are alternate options. If a carbapenem is used, addition of a second antipseudomonal agent is recommended.

Central Nervous System Infections

Bacterial brain abscesses are uncommon but may develop following head trauma or a neurosurgical procedure, as a result of hematogenous spread, or from an adjacent site of infection, such as a severe ear infection. Aspiration and drainage of the infection and treatment with ceftazidime with or without an aminoglycoside is recommended. Intravenous ciprofloxacin, aztreonam, or a carbapenem are alternate choices, as well as the addition of a second antipseudomonal agent.

References

1. Garau J, Gomez L: *Pseudomonas aeruginosa* pneumonia. *Curr Opin Infect Dis* 2003;16:135-143.

2. Burgess DS, Hall RG, Hardin TC: In vitro evaluation of the activity of two doses of levofloxacin alone and in combination with other agents against *Pseudomonas aeruginosa*. *Diagn Microbiol Infect Dis* 2003;46:131-137.

3. Ohl CA, Pollack M: Infections due to *Pseudomonas* species and related organisms. In: Braunwald E, Fauci AS, Kasper DL, et al, eds. *Harrison's Principles of Internal Medicine*, 15th ed. New York, NY, McGraw-Hill, 2001, pp 963-970.

4. Kollef MH: Gram-negative bacterial resistance: evolving patterns and treatment paradigms. *Clin Infect Dis* 2005;40(suppl 2):S85-S88.

5. Livermore DM: Multiple mechanisms of antimicrobial resistance in *Pseudomonas aeruginosa*: our worst nightmare? *Clin Infect Dis* 2002;34:634-640.

6. Allen L, Dockrell DH, Pattery T, et al: Pyocyanin production by *Pseudomonas aeruginosa* induces neutrophil apoptosis and impairs neutrophil-mediated host defenses in vivo. *J Immunol* 2005;174:3643-3649.

7. Van Delden C, Iglewski BH: Cell-to-cell signaling and *Pseudomonas aeruginosa* infections. *Emerg Infect Dis* 1998;4: 551-560.

8. Linden PK, Kusne S, Coley K, et al: Use of parenteral colistin for the treatment of serious infection due to antimicrobial-resistant *Pseudomonas aeruginosa. Clin Infect Dis* 2003;37:154-160.

9. Poole K: Aminoglycoside resistance in *Pseudomonas aeruginosa. Antimicrob Agents Chemother* 2005;49:479-487.

10. Poole K, Srikumar R: Multidrug efflux in *Pseudomonas aeruginosa*: components, mechanisms and clinical significance. *Curr Top Med Chem* 2001;1:59-71.

11. Jaffar-Bandjee MC, Lazdunski A, Bally M, et al: Production of elastase, exotoxin A, and alkaline protease in sputa during pulmonary exacerbation of cystic fibrosis in patients chronically infected by *Pseudomonas aeruginosa. J Clin Microbiol* 1995;33:924-929.

12. Roy-Burman A, Savel RH, Racine S, et al: Type III protein secretion is associated with death in lower respiratory and systemic *Pseudomonas aeruginosa* infections. *J Infect Dis* 2001;183: 1767-1774.

13. Spencer RC: Predominant pathogens found in the European Prevalence of Infection in Intensive Care Study. *Eur J Clin Microbiol Infect Dis* 1996;15:281-285.

14. Jones RN: Resistance patterns among nosocomial pathogens: trends over the past few years. *Chest* 2001;119:397S-404S.

15. Rennie RP, Jones RN, Mutnick AH, SENTRY Program Study Group (North America): Occurrence and antimicrobial susceptibility patterns of pathogens isolated from skin and soft tissue infections: report from the SENTRY Antimicrobial Surveillance Program (United States and Canada, 2000). *Diagn Microbiol Infect Dis* 2003;45:287-293.

16. Diekema DJ, Pfaller MA, Jones RN, et al: Survey of bloodstream infections due to gram-negative bacilli: frequency of occurrence and antimicrobial susceptibility of isolates collected in the United States, Canada, and Latin America for the SENTRY Antimicrobial Surveillance Program, 1997. *Clin Infect Dis* 1999;29: 595-607.

17. Gordon KA, Jones RN, SENTRY Participant Groups (Europe, Latin America, North America): Susceptibility patterns of orally

administered antimicrobials among urinary tract infection pathogens from hospitalized patients in North America: comparison report to Europe and Latin America. Results from the SENTRY Antimicrobial Surveillance Program (2000). *Diagn Microbiol Infect Dis* 2003;45:295-301.

18. National Nosocomial Infections Surveillance (NNIS) System: National Nosocomial Infections Surveillance (NNIS) System Report: data summary from January 1992 through June 2004, issued October 2004. *Am J Infect Control* 2004;32:470-485.

19. Centers for Disease Control and Prevention: Epidemiologic notes and reports *Pseudomonas aeruginosa* peritonitis attributed to a contaminated iodophor solution—Georgia. *MMWR Morb Mortal Wkly Rep* 1982;31:197-198.

20. Moore JE, Heaney N, Millar BC, et al: Incidence of *Pseudomonas aeruginosa* in recreational and hydrotherapy pools. *Commun Dis Public Health* 2002;5:23-26.

21. Centers for Disease Control and Prevention: Notice to readers: *Pseudomonas aeruginosa* infections associated with defective bronchoscopes. *MMWR Morb Mortal Wkly Rep* 2002;51:190.

22. Fraser TG, Reiner S, Malczynski M, et al: Multidrug-resistant *Pseudomonas aeruginosa* cholangitis after endoscopic retrograde cholangiopancreatography: failure of routine endoscope cultures to prevent an outbreak. *Infect Control Hosp Epidemiol* 2004;25:856-859.

23. Landman D, Quale JM, Mayorga D, et al: Citywide clonal outbreak of multiresistant *Acinetobacter baumannii* and *Pseudomonas aeruginosa* in Brooklyn, NY: the preantibiotic era has returned. *Arch Intern Med* 2002;162:1515-1520.

24. Dupeyron C, Mangeney N, Sedrati L, et al: Rapid emergence of quinolone resistance in cirrhotic patients treated with norfloxacin to prevent spontaneous bacterial peritonitis. *Antimicrob Agents Chemother* 1994;38:340-344.

25. Zervos MJ, Hershberger E, Nicolau DP, et al: Relationship between fluoroquinolone use and changes in susceptibility to fluoroquinolones of selected pathogens in 10 United States teaching hospitals, 1991-2000. *Clin Infect Dis* 2003;37:1643-1648.

26. Walsh FM, Amyes SG: Microbiology and drug resistance mechanisms of fully resistant pathogens. *Curr Opin Microbiol* 2004;7:439-444.

27. Karlowsky JA, Jones ME, Thornsberry C, et al: Stable antimicrobial susceptibility rates for clinical isolates of *Pseudomonas aeruginosa* from the 2001-2003 tracking resistance in the United States today surveillance studies. *Clin Infect Dis* 2005;40(suppl 2):S89-S98.

28. Siegman-Igra Y, Ravona R, Primerman H, et al: *Pseudomonas aeruginosa* bacteremia: an analysis of 123 episodes, with particular emphasis on the effect of antibiotic therapy. *Int J Infect Dis* 1998;2:211-215.

29. Mendelson MH, Gurtman A, Szabo S, et al: *Pseudomonas aeruginosa* bacteremia in patients with AIDS. *Clin Infect Dis* 1994;18:886-895.

30. Bergen GA, Shelhamer JH: Pulmonary infiltrates in the cancer patient. New approaches to an old problem. *Infect Dis Clin North Am* 1996;10:297-325.

31. Carmeli Y, Troillet N, Karchmer AW, et al: Health and economic outcomes of antibiotic resistance in *Pseudomonas aeruginosa*. *Arch Intern Med* 1999;159:1127-1132.

32. Giamarellou H: Prescribing guidelines for severe *Pseudomonas infections*. *J Antimicrob Chemother* 2002;49:229-233.

33. Bowton DL: Nosocomial pneumonia in the ICU—year 2000 and beyond. *Chest* 1999;115(3 suppl):28S-33S.

34. Beers MH, Berkow R, eds: Bacterial diseases. In: *The Merck Manual of Diagnosis and Therapy*, 17th ed. Whitehouse Station, NJ, Merck Research Laboratories, 1999, pp 1147-1209.

35. Kang C-I, Kim S-H, Kim H-B, et al: *Pseudomonas aeruginosa* bacteremia: risk factors for mortality and influence of delayed receipt of effective antimicrobial therapy on clinical outcome. *Clin Infect Dis* 2003;37:745-751.

36. Osmon S, Ward S, Fraser VJ, et al: Hospital mortality for patients with bacteremia due to *Staphylococcus aureus* or *Pseudomonas aeruginosa*. *Chest* 2004;125:607-616.

37. Kumar D, Cattral MS, Robicsek A, et al: Outbreak of *Pseudomonas aeruginosa* by multiple organ transplantation from a common donor. *Transplantation* 2003;75:1053-1055.

38. Berra L, De Marchi L, Yu ZX, et al: Endotracheal tubes coated with antiseptics decrease bacterial colonization of the ventilator circuits, lungs, and endotracheal tube. *Anesthesiology* 2004;100:1446-1456.

39.   FitzSimmons SC: The changing epidemiology of cystic fibrosis. *Curr Probl Pediatr* 1994;24:171-179.

40.   Mohr JF, Wanger A, Rex JH: Pharmacokinetic/pharmacodynamic modeling can help guide targeted antimicrobial therapy for nosocomial gram-negative infections in critically ill patients. *Diagn Microbiol Infect Dis* 2004;48:125-130.

41.   Zelenitsky SA, Harding GK, Sun S, et al: Treatment and outcome of *Pseudomonas aeruginosa* bacteremia: an antibiotic pharmacodynamic analysis. *J Antimicrob Chemother* 2003;52:668-674.

42.   Lynch JP 3rd: Hospital-acquired pneumonia: risk factors, microbiology, and treatment. *Chest* 2001;119(suppl 2):373S-384S.

43.   Hanna H, Afif C, Alakech B, et al: Central venous catheter-related bacteremia due to gram-negative bacilli: significance of catheter removal in preventing relapse. *Infect Control Hosp Epidemiol* 2004;25:646-649.

44.   Safdar N, Handelsman J, Maki DG: Does combination antimicrobial therapy reduce mortality in gram-negative bacteremia? A meta-analysis. *Lancet Infect Dis* 2004;4:519-527.

45.   Chamot E, Boffi El Amari E, et al: Effectiveness of combination antimicrobial therapy for *Pseudomonas aeruginosa* bacteremia. *Antimicrob Agents Chemother* 2003;47:2756-2764.

46.   Jacobs RA, Guglielmo BJ: Anti-infective chemotherapeutic and antibiotic agents. In: Tierney LM Jr, McPhee SJ, Papadakis MA, eds. *Current Medical Diagnosis and Treatment*, 43rd ed. New York, NY, McGraw Hill/Appleton & Lange Medical Books/McGraw-Hill, 2004, pp 1486-1526.

47.   Erasmo AA, Crisostomo AC, Yan LN, et al: Randomized comparison of piperacillin/tazobactam versus imipenem/cilastatin in the treatment of patients with intra-abdominal infection. *Asian J Surg* 2004;27:227-235.

48.   West M, Boulanger BR, Fogarty C, et al: Levofloxacin compared with imipenem/cilastatin followed by ciprofloxacin in adult patients with nosocomial pneumonia: a multicenter, prospective, randomized, open-label study. *Clin Ther* 2003;25:485-506.

49.   Sobieszczyk ME, Furuya EY, Hay CM, et al: Combination therapy with polymyxin B for the treatment of multidrug-resistant gram-negative respiratory tract infections. *J Antimicrob Chemother* 2004;54:566-569.

50.   Moss RB: Long-term benefits of inhaled tobramycin in adolescent patients with cystic fibrosis. *Chest* 2002;121:55-63.

51.   Hodson ME, Gallagher CG, Govan JR: A randomised clinical trial of nebulised tobramycin or colistin in cystic fibrosis. *Eur Respir J* 2002;20:658-664.

52.   Grossman RF: The role of fluoroquinolones in respiratory tract infections. *J Antimicrob Chemother* 1997;40(suppl A):59-62.

53.   Madoff LC: Infectious complications of bites and burns. In: Braunwald E, Fauci AS, Kasper DL, et al, eds. *Harrison's Principles of Internal Medicine*, 15th ed. New York, NY, McGraw-Hill, 2001, pp 817-825.

54.   Ozkiris A, Evereklioglu C, Esel D, et al: The efficacy of piperacillin/tazobactam in experimental *Pseudomonas aeruginosa* endophthalmitis: a histopathological and microbiological evaluation. *Curr Eye Res* 2005;30:13-19.

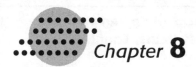

Chapter 8

Prevention and Control of Antimicrobial-Resistant Bacteria

Antimicrobial resistance significantly affects health care by the severity of diseases, the mortality and morbidity for some infections, and the costs of treatment. According to data gathered by the Centers for Disease Control and Prevention (CDC), nearly 2 million hospitalized patients acquire a nosocomial infection each year.

About 90,000 of those patients die each year as a result of their infection. More than 70% of the bacteria that cause nosocomial infections are resistant to one or more of the antibiotics commonly used to treat them, and patients infected with antimicrobial-resistant organisms are likely to have longer hospital stays and require treatment with second- and third-choice drugs that may be less effective. These drugs also have more adverse effects and cost more.[1]

Prevention and control of antimicrobial resistance require a commitment to two policies: infection control measures that limit the spread of resistant organisms and judicious use of antimicrobials. Involvement of prescribers, patients, and health-care administrators is essential to implement efforts to combat antimicrobial resistance.

Physicians need to understand that their prescribing actions have a cumulative impact on patterns of resistance. A study by members of the CDC Campaign to Prevent Antimicrobial Resistance assessed clinicians' perceptions of antimicrobial resistance.[2] The study found that clini-

Table 8-1: Responses of 10,780 People* to Survey Items, FoodNet Population Survey

Survey Item

In the past 4 weeks, have you taken any antibiotic medicine?

When I have a cold, I should take antibiotics to prevent getting a more serious illness.

When I get a cold, antibiotics help me to get better more quickly.

By the time I am sick enough to talk to or visit a doctor because of a cold, I usually expect a prescription for antibiotics.

Are you aware of any health dangers to yourself or other people associated with taking antibiotics?

*Values are numbers of persons who answered the questions or statements. Percentages are based on weighted population data.
(From Vanden Eng[5])

cians are significantly more likely to perceive antimicrobial resistance as a problem nationally rather than a problem in their own community, institution, or practice.

Studies have shown that patients' expectations or physicians' perceptions of those expectations affect prescribing behavior.[3,4] Educational interventions directed at patients can not only increase their knowledge of appropriate antibiotic use, but can also decrease the frequency with which clinicians prescribe antibiotics inappropriately.

A telephone survey by the Foodborne Diseases Active Surveillance Network (FoodNet) gathered data on con-

Yes/Agree	No/Disagree	Unsure	%Yes
1,255	9,485	N/A	12.0
2,544	7,638	538	27.4
3,053	6,758	896	32.2
4,812	4,954	911	47.6
4,860	5,749	164	41.9

sumer attitudes about use of antibiotics.[5] Questions involved consumers' knowledge, attitudes, and practices of antibiotic use (Table 8-1). Demographics showed that people of higher education and income were more likely to have better access to health care and to have medical insurance. They were also more likely to use antibiotics.

Health-care administrators need to be convinced that actions designed to improve antimicrobial use and resistance are needed and cost-effective. Administrative support is important for antimicrobial monitoring programs to improve use of antimicrobials.[6]

Infection Control

The World Health Organization (WHO) recommends a global strategy for infection control in health-care facilities.[7] According to the WHO, the essential elements of an infection control program are basic infection control measures, education of health-care workers, surveillance of hospital-associated infections, and appropriate legislation.

The Hospital Infection Control Practices Advisory Committee (HICPAC) of the CDC formulated Guidelines for Isolation Precautions in Hospitals[8] with two levels of precautions: standard precautions, which apply to the care of all patients in hospitals, regardless of their diagnosis, and transmission-based precautions, which are for patients with known or suspected infection by epidemiologically important pathogens. Pathogens from this type of patient involve airborne, droplet, or contact transmission.

Standard Precautions

Standard precautions are designed to reduce the risk of transmission of bloodborne pathogens and pathogens from moist body substances.[9] Standard precautions apply to blood, body fluids, secretions, excretions, mucous membranes, and nonintact skin.[8] Infection control measures include handwashing; various means of barrier protection; proper handling of patient-care equipment, linens, and articles; patient placement and transport; cleaning of dishes, glasses, cups, and eating utensils; and routine and terminal cleaning of patient rooms.

Handwashing. Handwashing is the most important way to reduce the risk of transmitting organisms from patient to patient, from one site to another on a patient, or from personnel to patients. Hands should be washed before and after direct contact with patients, as well as after contact with blood, body fluids, secretions, excretions, or contaminated items, even if gloves are worn. Hands should also be washed after gloves are removed and between

Table 8-2: Potential Benefits of Alcohol-based Sinkless Hand Rubs

	Soap and water handwashing	Alcohol hand rub
Time required	30-120 seconds	10-30 seconds
Efficacy in degerming	Good to very good	Excellent
Acceptance by personnel	Historically poor	Good to excellent

(from Weinstein[10])

patient contacts or between procedures on the same patient to prevent cross-contamination on the body.

Despite its importance, handwashing remains the most frequently neglected infection control measure in hospitals. Two main factors contribute to handwashing noncompliance: the time it takes, which is estimated to be up to 90 minutes per work shift, and the irritation it causes to the skin.[10]

Alcohol-based hand rubs have gained acceptance to improve compliance in hand hygiene. The CDC Guidelines for Hand Hygiene in Health-Care Settings indicate that alcohol-based hand rubs containing emollients are less irritating to the skin than soaps.[11] It addition, it takes less time to use hand rubs and it is unnecessary to wash or rinse hands after using them (Table 8-2). However, because these products do not kill spores, hands should be washed with soap and water after contact with patients infected with *Clostridium difficile*. Finally, compliance with the CDC hand hygiene guidelines is now one of the Joint Commission for the Accreditation of Healthcare Organizations (JCAHO) National Patient Safety Goals.

Gloves and Gowns. Gloves are worn to prevent contamination of hands when touching blood, body fluids, secretions, excretions, and contaminated items. Clean gloves should be put on before touching mucous membranes of areas of open skin. Gloves should be changed between procedures on the same patient after contact with potentially infectious material. Gloves should be removed immediately after use, and hands should be washed between patient contacts. Wearing gloves does not replace the need for handwashing.

The use of gowns is primarily to protect personnel by preventing contamination of clothing with infectious organisms during blood and body fluid exposures. Adherence to the Occupational Safety and Health Administration (OSHA) bloodborne pathogens rule makes wearing of gowns and protective apparel mandatory under specific circumstances. When splashes or spray of blood, body fluids, secretions, and excretions are likely to occur, a gown, mask, and eye protection should be worn.

Patient-care Equipment and Linens. Used patient care equipment and linens that have been in contact with blood, body fluids, secretions, and excretions should be handled in such a way as to prevent exposure to skin and mucous membranes, contamination of clothing, or transfer of organisms to other patients, patient-care personnel, or the environment. Reusable equipment must be properly disinfected and processed before reuse and disposable items must be properly discarded.

Environmental Control. High standards of environmental cleaning play an important role in the prevention of outbreaks of infectious organisms in the hospital.[12] Hospital procedures should be in place for routine care, cleaning, and disinfection of environmental surfaces, as well as terminal disinfection and cleaning of rooms between patients.

Patient Placement and Transport

Ideally, patients infected with highly transmissible pathogens should be placed in private rooms with handwashing and toilet facilities to minimize potential for transfer of infectious organisms. Also, patients who have limited ability to comply with infection control precautions—infants, children, and patients with altered mental status—should be in private rooms.

When a private room is not available, patients infected with the same organism can usually share a room. This cohorting of patients is often used during outbreaks or when there is a shortage of rooms. When an infected patient shares a room with a noninfected person, consultation with an infection control officer is recommended to make a careful selection of roommates. Patients, personnel, and visitors need to take appropriate precautions to prevent the spread of the infectious organism.

When an infected patient is transported, he or she should wear barrier protection such as masks and impervious dressings to reduce the opportunity for transmission of infectious organisms. People in the area to which the patient is being transported should be notified of the required precautions, and the patients themselves should be advised of ways to prevent transmission of their infectious organisms.

Patient-care Equipment, Linens, and Articles. Special handling of used patient-care equipment and articles may be required, depending on the likelihood of contamination with infective material, the ability of sharp materials to cause injury, the epidemiologic features of the infective pathogen, and its environmental stability. Used sharps must be deposited in puncture-resistant containers. Two bags may be used for items contaminated with particularly infectious organisms or when the outside of the first bag becomes contaminated while articles are being placed in it.

Reusable equipment should be sterilized or disinfected, following hospital policy and manufacturer's recommendations. Hospital policy also guides handling of contaminated linens. Reusable eating utensils, dishes, cups, and glasses do not require special precautions because the detergents and hot water in hospital dishwashers are sufficient to decontaminate such items.

Occupational Health and Bloodborne Pathogens

For protection of health-care workers, used needles should never be recapped, bent, or broken by hand. Disposable syringes, needles, scalpels, and other sharp items should be placed in puncture-resistant containers provided for them and located as close as possible to the areas where they are used.

Mouthpieces, resuscitation bags, or other ventilation devices should be accessible in areas where resuscitation might be necessary and should be used preferentially to mouth-to-mouth resuscitation.

Transmission-based Precautions

Transmission-based precautions are designed for patients with documented or suspected infections or colonization with highly transmissible or epidemiologically important pathogens. For these patients, special precautions are needed in addition to standard precautions.

The main routes of transmission of organisms in hospitals are contact, droplet, airborne, and common vehicle.[9,13] Contact transmission is the most frequent mode of transmission of nosocomial infections and is also the only mode of transmission thought to be relevant to the transmission of resistant bacteria, with the exception of *Mycobacterium tuberculosis*.[9]

Contact Transmission. Direct contact involves physical transfer of an organism by skin-to-skin contact between a susceptible host and an infected or colonized person. Indirect contact involves transmission from a contaminated object to a susceptible host. Contaminated instruments, dressings, linens, and environmental surfaces can be sources of indirect contact transmission, as are gloves that are not changed or hands not washed between patient contacts.[8]

Contact precautions include wearing gloves when entering a room, changing gloves after contact with infective material, and removing gloves and washing hands with an antimicrobial or antiseptic agent before leaving the room. A gown should be worn if contact with the patient, infective material, or environmental surfaces is likely. The gown should be removed before a clinician leaves the room and should be properly discarded.[8]

Precautions should be maintained during transport of the patient. Dedicated use of noncritical patient-care equipment to a single patient is preferred; otherwise, shared equipment must be adequately cleaned and disinfected between uses.

Droplet Transmission. When a patient coughs, talks, or sneezes, droplets containing infective organisms are dispersed a short distance into the air and may be deposited on a host's conjunctivae, nasal mucosa, or mouth. Procedures such as bronchoscopy and suctioning may also spread droplets. To prevent transmission of infectious agents spread by droplets, the patient should have a private room. If a private room is not available, cohorting is preferable, and if this is not possible, a space of at least 3 feet should be maintained between the infected patient and other patients or visitors. Personnel and visitors should wear a mask when within 3 feet of the patient, and the patient should wear a mask, if possible, when transported.[8]

Airborne Transmission. Airborne transmission differs from droplet transmission in that the infective agent is carried on dust particles or as nuclei of evaporated droplets that remain suspended in the air for long periods. A private room with handwashing and toilet facilities should be used and special air handling and ventilation are required to prevent airborne particle transmission. If a private room is not available, cohorting is recommended with a patient who has the same active infection, but no infection with additional organisms. The door to the room should be kept closed. Any person entering the room should wear a respiratory mask designed for airborne particles, and if the patient must be transported, the patient must wear a similar mask.[8]

Table 8-3: Clinical Syndromes Warranting Additional Empiric Precautions

Clinical Syndrome or Condition*	Empiric Precautions
Diarrhea	
Acute diarrhea with a likely infectious cause	Contact
Diarrhea in an adult with a history of recent antibiotic use	Contact
Meningitis	Droplet
Rash or exanthems, generalized, etiology unknown	
Petechial/ecchymotic with fever	Droplet
Vesicular	Airborne and contact
Maculopapular with coryza and fever	Airborne
Respiratory infections	
Cough/fever/pulmonary infiltrate	Airborne
Paroxysmal or severe persistent cough during periods of pertussis activity	Droplet

Clinical Syndromes Requiring Transmission-based Precautions

Because the risk of nosocomial transmission may be highest before a definitive diagnosis can be made, certain clinical syndromes warrant transmission-based precautions. For patients with diarrhea, meningitis, rashes of unknown etiology, respiratory infections, and skin and wound infections, additional empiric precautions are warranted. Patients with a history of infection or colonization with multidrug-resistant organisms also warrant enhanced precautions to prevent the potential transmission of in-

Clinical Syndrome or Condition*	Empiric Precautions
Respiratory infections, particularly bronchiolitis and croup, in infants and young children	Contact
Risk of multidrug-resistant microorganisms	
History of infection or colonization with multidrug-resistant organisms	Contact
Skin, wound, or urinary tract infection in a patient with a recent hospital	Contact
or nursing home stay where multidrug-resistant organisms are prevalent	Contact
Skin or wound infection	
Abscess or draining wound that cannot be covered	Contact

* Infection control professionals are encouraged to modify or adapt this table according to local conditions. (Modified from Garner[8])

fectious agents (Table 8-3). Immunocompromised patients are generally at increased risk for infections from both endogenous and exogenous sources and may also warrant additional precautions.

Multidrug-resistant Organisms

Preventing the spread of multidrug-resistant (MDR) organisms such as vancomycin-resistant enterococci (VRE), methicillin-resistant *Staphylococcus aureus* (MRSA), and *Acinetobacter* is particularly important, because treatment for these organisms is limited. Patients previously colonized or infected with VRE can remain

Table 8-4: Recommendations for Preventing Intravascular Catheter-related Infections

- Educate and train health-care providers who insert and maintain catheters.

- Use maximum sterile barrier precautions during central venous catheter insertion.

- Use a 2% chlorhexidine preparation for skin antisepsis.

- Avoid routine replacement of central venous catheters.

- Use antiseptic/antibiotic impregnated short-term central venous catheters if the rate of infection is high despite adherence to the other strategies.

(From O'Grady[18])

colonized for long periods. If they are readmitted to the hospital, there is a risk of transmission of the organism. Therefore, institutions should have a mechanism in place to identify these patients and place them in isolation. The use of gowns in addition to gloves has been shown to decrease the nosocomial transmission of resistant organisms such as VRE.[14,15]

Surveillance

A survey of members of the Infectious Diseases Society of America Emerging Infections Network showed that most infectious disease experts approve the use of contact precautions for routine management of patients infected or colonized with MDR organisms.[16] Opinions are divided, however, on the usefulness of routine surveillance for managing such organisms.

Table 8-5: Major Recommendations for Prevention of Catheter-associated Urinary Tract Infections

- Educate personnel in correct techniques of catheter insertion and care.

- Catheterize only when necessary.

- Emphasize handwashing.

- Insert catheter using aseptic technique and sterile equipment.

- Secure catheter properly.

- Maintain closed sterile drainage.

- Obtain urine samples aseptically.

- Maintain unobstructed urine flow.

(From Wong[19])

A task force for the Society for Healthcare Epidemiology of America (SHEA) drafted a guide for preventing nosocomial transmission of MDR strains of *S aureus* and *Enterococcus*. The group concluded that active surveillance cultures are essential to identify the reservoir for the spread of MRSA and VRE infections and for infection control.[17] Despite these recommendations, active surveillance remains controversial.

Catheter-related Infections

The use of foreign devices, such as intravascular and urinary catheters, is associated with an increased risk of infection. Guidelines have been formulated for prevention of intravascular catheter-related infections[18] and for prevention of catheter-associated urinary tract infections[19]

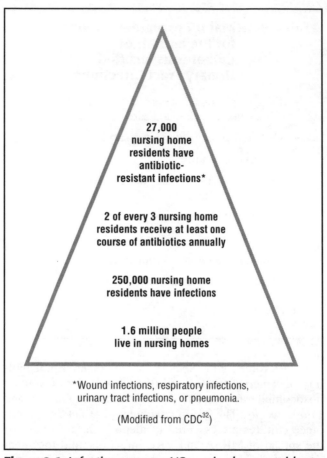

27,000
nursing home
residents have
antibiotic-
resistant infections*

2 of every 3 nursing home
residents receive at least one
course of antibiotics annually

250,000 nursing home
residents have infections

1.6 million people
live in nursing homes

*Wound infections, respiratory infections,
urinary tract infections, or pneumonia.

(Modified from CDC[32])

Figure 8-1: Infections among US nursing home residents.

(Table 8-4 and Table 8-5). Education of personnel who insert catheters and the use of aseptic technique are critical to reduce the likelihood of infection.

The catheter and site for peripheral venous catheters should be changed no more frequently than every 72 to

96 hours, at which time a new dressing should be applied. In addition, the dressing should be changed whenever it becomes loose, soiled, or damp.

Peripheral arterial catheters and central venous catheters should not be routinely replaced. The same conditions apply to changing the dressing as with peripheral venous catheter dressings.[18] Urinary catheters should be inserted only when necessary and left in place only for as long as necessary.[19]

Prevention of Infection in Long-term Care Facilities

Patients in long-term care facilities often have host defense deficits that predispose them to infection, including thinning skin, urinary retention, and diminished ability to clear their airways.[20] Underlying diseases such as diabetes mellitus and cancer, as well as alteration in mental status, also increase these patients' risk of infection. Incontinence, use of indwelling urinary catheters, lack of mobility, and use of steroids and antibiotics further predispose many long-term-care patients to infection (Figure 8-1).

As in acute care hospitals, active surveillance is recommended in long-term care facilities to collect data and detect infection.[20] Standard and transmission-based precautions apply to long-term-care facilities. Handwashing is the most important infection control measure, just as it is in the hospital.

Resident health programs emphasize vaccination of elderly people with tetanus and diphtheria as well as pneumococcal and influenza immunizations. Monitoring of employee health is another important factor in the transmission of pathogens. Education of employees in infection control principles and policies is an essential part of infection control in long-term-care facilities.

Appropriate Use of Antibiotics

Multiple studies have shown links between antimicrobial use and the development of antimicrobial resistance.

Important findings from studies include the following: (1) changes in antimicrobial usage are paralleled by changes in the prevalence of resistance; (2) antimicrobial resistance is more prevalent in nosocomial strains than in those from community-acquired infections; (3) during outbreaks of nosocomial infections, patients infected with resistant strains are more likely than control patients to have received prior antibiotics; (4) areas within hospitals that have the highest rates of resistance also have the highest rates of antibiotic use; (5) and increasing the duration of patient exposure to antimicrobials increases the likelihood of colonization with resistant organisms.[9]

Because few new antimicrobials are in development, controlling antimicrobial resistance is vital to preserving the efficacy of the antimicrobials that are available (Figure 1-1). Judicious use of antimicrobials is a key element in controlling resistance.

A multidisciplinary group of experts were joined by representatives from the pharmaceutical industry, the JCAHO, and appropriate federal agencies to draft a model that hospitals might use to develop a plan to reduce antimicrobial resistance.[21] The workshop formulated five strategic goals to optimize the prophylactic, empiric, and therapeutic use of antibiotics in the hospital: (1) optimize choice and duration of prophylactic antibiotic therapy; (2) optimize choice and duration of empiric antibiotic therapy; (3) improve antibiotic prescribing practices by educational and administrative means; (4) establish a system to monitor and provide feedback on the occurrence and impact of antibiotic resistance; (5) and define and implement institutional or health-care delivery-system guidelines for important types of antibiotic use. Development of hospital policies should be based on local resistance data and antibiotic usage patterns with input from regional and state departments of health as well as from national organizations.[9]

Appropriate antimicrobial stewardship includes both limiting the use of inappropriate agents and selecting the appropriate dosing and duration of antimicrobials to achieve optimal efficacy. Various measures have been recommended to improve antibiotic use, including formularies, cycling of antimicrobials, clinical practice guidelines, computer-assisted decision-making, and combination therapy.

Formularies

Many hospitals have formulary restrictions, but it is the patterns and volume of drug use that impact resistance.[22] Several important studies have shown that changes in antimicrobial formularies have an impact on antibiotic resistance.[23-25] Reduction in resistance of the target organisms, however, has often been accompanied by increases in resistance in other organisms.

A study at a Veterans Affairs medical center in 1995 assessed the effect of prescribing restrictions for cefotaxime (Claforan®), clindamycin (Cleocin®), and vancomycin (Vancocin®) in response to an increase in VRE infections.[24] Use of ampicillin/sulbactam (Unasyn®) or piperacillin/tazobactam (Zosyn®) was recommended in place of cephalosporins, and clindamycin use was restricted because of a concurrent outbreak of *Clostridium difficile*.

The changes resulted in reductions in the use of cefazolin (Ancef®, Kefzol®), ceftazidime (Ceptaz®, Fortaz®), imipenem (Primaxin®), and gentamicin (Garamycin®) as well as clindamycin, cefotaxime, and vancomycin. Significant reductions in the incidence of MRSA and ceftazidime-resistant *Klebsiella pneumoniae* ensued, but significant increases in infections by cefotaxime-resistant *Acinetobacter* also occurred.

At another hospital, formulary changes decreased the use of cephalosporins by 80%, which resulted in significant reductions in ceftazidime-resistant *Klebsiella* infections and colonization throughout the hospital.[25] These formulary changes, however, were accompanied by an increase in imipenem use and a 69% increase in infections caused by imipenem-resistant *P aeruginosa*.

A general recommendation suggested for formulary restrictions is to restrict antibiotics with high-resistance potential, such as third-generation cephalosporins, quinolones, and carbapenems, and replace them with antibiotics with low-resistance potential, such as cefepime (Maxipime®) or piperacillin/tazobactam. It is also suggested that clinicians in the outpatient setting use oral antibiotics with low-resistance potential, such as clindamycin, metronidazole (Flagyl®), doxycycline (Doryx®, Vibramycin®), and minocycline (Minocin®) in preference to antibiotics with high-resistance potential.[26] Use of narrow-spectrum antibiotics over broad-spectrum antibiotics is also advised.[27]

Cycling of Antimicrobials

Antimicrobial cycling is the scheduled removal of one specific antimicrobial or class of antimicrobials and substitution with another, with the aim of avoiding or reversing the development of antimicrobial resistance.[28] The duration of the switch may be determined on the basis of local resistance patterns or be a preset length of time.

This tactic has the potential to develop a new resistance problem, and clinicians might not comply with cycling restrictions. Clinician concerns over patient allergies, side effects, or consistency with national guidelines cause 10% to 50% of patients to be treated with antimicrobials other than the chosen substitute.[28] Cycling is most likely to be effective for limited periods in closed environments, such as ICUs,[10] but additional studies need to be conducted before the impact of antimicrobial cycling is clear.

Clinical Practice Guidelines

Many hospitals establish clinical practice guidelines. In a study of practices to improve antimicrobial use at 47 hospitals, clinical practice guidelines were reported at 33 of the hospitals (70%).[29] The guidelines were either criteria-

Table 8-6: Situations in Which Use of Vancomycin is Appropriate or Acceptable

- For treatment of serious infections caused by β-lactam-resistant gram-positive microorganisms.

- For treatment of infections caused by gram-positive microorganisms in patients who have serious allergies to β-lactam antimicrobials.

- When antibiotic-associated colitis fails to respond to metronidazole therapy or is severe and potentially life threatening.

- Prophylaxis, as recommended by the American Heart Association, for endocarditis after certain procedures in patients at high risk for endocarditis.

- Prophylaxis for major surgical procedures involving implantation of prosthetic materials or devices (eg, cardiac and vascular procedures and total hip replacement) at institutions that have a high rate of infections caused by MRSA or methicillin-resistant *S epidermidis*. A single dose of vancomycin administered immediately before surgery is sufficient unless the procedure lasts more than 6 hours, in which case the dose should be repeated. Prophylaxis should be discontinued after a maximum of two doses.

(From CDC[14])

based or diagnosis-based. Criteria-based guidelines describe appropriate vs inappropriate use for specific antimicrobials or groups of antimicrobials. Diagnosis-based guidelines describe treatment by syndrome or clinical condition.

Table 8-7: Situations in Which the Use of Vancomycin Should Be Discouraged

- Routine surgical prophylaxis other than for a patient with life-threatening allergy to β-lactam antibiotics.

- Empiric antimicrobial therapy for a febrile neutropenic patient, unless initial evidence indicates that the patient has an infection caused by gram-positive microorganisms (eg, at an inflamed exit site of a Hickman catheter) and the prevalence of infections caused by MRSA in the hospital is substantial.

- Treatment in response to a single blood culture positive for coagulase-negative staphylococcus, if other blood cultures taken during the same time frame are negative.

- Continued empiric use for presumed infections in patients whose cultures are negative for β-lactam-resistant gram-positive microorganisms.

The most common criteria-based guideline reported at 29 hospitals (62%) was for vancomycin. Teaching hospitals were significantly more likely than other hospitals to have clinical practice guidelines for vancomycin use and also for treatment of community-acquired pneumonia.

Vancomycin Guidelines

Because the use of vancomycin is associated with risk for infection and colonization with VRE, the Hospital Infection Control Practices Advisory Committee (HICPAC)

- Systemic or local (eg, antibiotic lock) prophylaxis for infection or colonization of indwelling central or peripheral intravascular catheters.

- Selective decontamination of digestive tract.

- Eradication of MRSA colonization.

- Primary treatment of antibiotic-associated colitis.

- Routine prophylaxis for very low-birthweight infants (<1,500 g or 3 lb 4 oz).

- Routine prophylaxis for patients on continuous ambulatory peritoneal dialysis or hemodialysis.

- Treatment of infections caused by β-lactam-sensitive gram-positive microorganisms in patients with renal failure.

- Use of vancomycin for topical application or irrigation.

(From CDC[14])

of the CDC developed recommendations for its use to prevent the spread of vancomycin resistance.[14] Although each hospital should develop its own appropriate guidelines, the HICPAC has specific recommendations for situations in which use of vancomycin is appropriate and in which its use should be discouraged (Table 8-6 and Table 8-7).

Computer-assisted Decision-Making

The use of computer decision-support programs shows promise for the appropriate selection of antimicrobials.

Computer-based order entry uses technology to provide the clinician with simple messages on suggested indications for, or local resistance patterns of, a selected antibiotic.[10] Some programs can integrate microbiology and laboratory tests into decision-making algorithms.[30]

Evans et al[30] developed and evaluated a computer decision-support program and found use of the program had many benefits. It led to a significant reduction in orders for drugs to which patients had reported allergies, excess drug dosages, and treatment with antibiotics to which the organism was resistant. Adverse events and the mean number of days of excessive drug dosage were also reduced.

Combination Therapy

Combination antimicrobial therapy is widely used for the treatment of seriously ill patients,[9] despite the lack of conclusive data that such therapy prevents emergence of antibiotic resistance. Mathematical models, however, do suggest that combination therapy is superior to single antibiotics in preventing resistance.[31]

CDC Campaign

The CDC launched a campaign to Prevent Antimicrobial Resistance in Healthcare Settings.[32] The campaign promotes four basic strategies for clinicians to use: prevent infection, diagnose and treat infection effectively, use antimicrobials wisely, and prevent transmission. The campaign includes information for preventing antimicrobial resistance among hospitalized patients, surgical patients, dialysis patients, and long-term care residents, each in a 12-step format. Educational material is also available for patients, including tips to prevent antimicrobial resistance for adult, surgical, and dialysis patients. The CDC Web site for this campaign to is http://www.cdc.gov/drugresistance/healthcare/default.htm.

References

1. Infectious Diseases Society of America report: Bad bugs, no drugs. July 2004; page 3. Available at: http://www.fda.gov/ohrms/dockets/04s0233/04s-0233-c000005-03-IDSA-vol1.pdf. Accessed June 10, 2005.

2. Gibl . TB, Sinkowitz-Cochran RL, Harris PL, et al: Clinicians' perceptions of the problem of antimicrobial resistance in health care facilities. *Arch Intern Med* 2004;164:1662-1668.

3. Bauchner H, Pelton SI, Klein JO: Parents, physicians, and antibiotic use. *Pediatrics* 1999;103:395-401.

4. Mangione-Smith R, McGlynn EA, Elliott MN, et al: Parent expectations for antibiotics, physician-parent communication, and satisfaction. *Arch Pediatr Adolesc Med* 2001;155:800-806.

5. Vanden Eng J, Marcus R, Hadler JL, et al: Consumer attitudes and use of antibiotics. *Emerg Infect Dis* 2003;9:1128-1135.

6. McGowan JE Jr: Minimizing antimicrobial resistance: the key role of the infectious diseases physician. *Clin Infect Dis* 2004;38:939-942.

7. Lazzari S. Allegranzi B, Concia E: Making hospitals safer: the need for a global strategy for infection control in health care settings. *World Hosp Health Serv* 2004;40:32,34,36-42.

8. Garner JS: Guideline for isolation precautions in hospitals. The Hospital Infection Control Practices Advisory Committee. *Infect Control Hosp Epidemiol* 1996;17:53-80.

9. Shlaes DM, Gerding DN, John JF Jr, et al: Society for Healthcare Epidemiology of America and Infectious Diseases Society of America Joint Committee on the Prevention of Antimicrobial Resistance: guidelines for the prevention of antimicrobial resistance in hospitals. *Infect Control Hosp Epidemiol* 1997;18:275-291.

10. Weinstein RA: Controlling antimicrobial resistance in hospitals: infection control and use of antibiotics. *Emerg Infect Dis* 2001;7:188-192.

11. Centers for Disease Control and Prevention: Guideline for hand hygiene in health-care settings. *MMWR Morb Mortal Wkly Rep* 2002;51:1-56.

12. Denton M, Wilcox MH, Parnell P, et al: Role of environmental cleaning in controlling an outbreak of *Acinetobacter*

225

baumannii on a neurosurgical intensive care unit. *J Hosp Infect* 2004;56:106-110.

13. Bolyard EA, Tablan OC, Williams WW, et al: Guideline for infection control in healthcare personnel, 1998 Hospital Infection Control Practices Advisory Committee. *Infect Control Hosp Epidemiol* 1998;19:407-463.

14. Centers for Disease Control and Prevention: Recommendations for preventing the spread of vancomycin resistance. *MMWR Morb Mortal Wkly Rep* 1995;44(RR-12):1-13.

15. Srinivasan A, Song X, Ross T, et al: A prospective study to determine whether cover gowns in addition to gloves decreases nosocomial transmission of vancomycin-resistant enterococci in an intensive care unit. *Infect Control Hosp Epidemiol* 2002;23: 424-428.

16. Sunenshine RH, Liedtke LA, Fridkin SK, et al: Management of inpatients colonized or infected with antimicrobial-resistant bacteria in hospitals in the United States. *Infect Control Hosp Epidemiol* 2005;26:138-143.

17. Muto CA, Jernigan JA, Ostrowsky BE, et al: SHEA guideline for preventing nosocomial transmission of multidrug-resistant strains of *Staphylococcus aureus* and enterococcus. *Infect Control Hosp Epidemiol* 2003;24:362-386.

18. O'Grady NP, Alexander M, Dellinger EP, et al: Guidelines for the prevention of intravascular catheter-related infections. Centers for Disease Control and Prevention. *MMWR Recomm Rep* 2002;51(RR-10):1-29.

19. Wong ES: Guideline for prevention of catheter-associated urinary tract infections. *Am J Infect Control* 1983;11:28-36.

20. Smith PW, Rusnak PG: Infection prevention and control in the long-term-care facility. SHEA Long-Term-Care Command and APIC Guidelines Committee position paper. Inf*ect Control Hosp Epidemiol* 1997;18:831-849.

21. Goldmann DA, Weinstein RA, Wenzel RP, et al: Strategies to prevent and control the emergence and spread of antimicrobial-resistant microorganisms in hospitals. A challenge to hospital leadership. *JAMA* 1996;275:234-240.

22. Polk RE: Antimicrobial formularies: can they minimize antimicrobial resistance? *Am J Health Syst Pharm* 2003;60(10 suppl 1): S16-S19.

23.   White AC Jr, Atmar RL, Wilson J, et al: Effects of requiring prior authorization for selected antimicrobials: expenditures, susceptibilities, and clinical outcomes. *Clin Infect Dis* 1997;25:230-239.

24.   Landman D, Chockalingam M, Quale JM: Reduction in the incidence of methicillin-resistant Staphylococcus aureus and ceftazidime-resistant *Klebsiella pneumoniae* following changes in a hospital antibiotic formulary. *Clin Infect Dis* 1999;28:1062-1066.

25.   Rahal JJ, Urban C, Segal-Maurer S: Nosocomial antibiotic resistance in multiple gram-negative species: experience at one hospital with squeezing the resistance balloon at multiple sites. *Clin Infect Dis* 2002;34:499-503.

26.   Cunha BA: Strategies to control antibiotic resistance. *Semin Respir Infect* 2002;17:250-258.

27.   Kollef MH, Fraser VJ: Antibiotic resistance in the intensive care unit. *Ann Intern Med* 2001;134:298-314.

28.   Fridkin SK: Routine cycling of antimicrobial agents as an infection-control measure. *Clin Infect Dis* 2003;36:1438-1444.

29.   Lawton RM, Fridkin SK, Gaynes RP, et al: Practices to improve antimicrobial use at 47 US hospitals: the status of the 1997 SHEA/IDSA position paper recommendations. Society for Healthcare Epidemiology of America/Infectious Diseases Society of America. *Infect Control Hosp Epidemiol* 2000;21:256-259.

30.   Evans RS, Pestotnik SL, Classen DC, et al: A computer-assisted management program for antibiotics and other antiinfective agents. *N Engl J Med* 1998;338:232-238.

31.   Bonhoeffer S, Lipsitch M, Levin BR: Evaluating treatment protocols to prevent antibiotic resistance. *Proc Natl Acad Sci USA* 1997;94:12106-12111.

32.   Centers for Disease Control and Prevention: Campaign to prevent antimicrobial resistance in healthcare settings. Available at: http://www.cdc.gov/drugresistance/healthcare/default.htm. Accessed June 14, 2005.

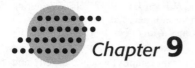 *Chapter* **9**

Future Antibiotic Armamentarium

T he research and development of new antimicrobials are expensive and time-consuming processes. Bringing a new antibiotic to the market can take 10 years or more and an investment in excess of $1 billion.[1] Despite a great need for antimicrobials with a novel mechanism of action to reduce resistance, only a few new antibiotics are in the late stages of development. Among these are tigecycline (Tygacil™), which is a recently approved glycylcycline; telavancin and dalbavancin, which are glycopeptides; and doripenem, which is a new carbapenem.

Tigecycline

Although tetracyclines have been in clinical use for more than 50 years, the widespread emergence of bacterial resistance has limited the effectiveness of this class of antibiotics.[2-4] Tigecycline is a novel, broad-spectrum, intravenous (IV) antimicrobial, the first of a new class of antibiotics, called glycylcyclines. Developed specifically to overcome tetracycline resistance, it has gained FDA approval for the treatment of complicated skin and soft-tissue infections and intra-abdominal infections, and is currently being evaluated for the treatment of community-acquired respiratory tract infections.[5-7] It recently received Food and Drug Administration (FDA) approval. Tigecycline is a minocycline derivative that has activity against a broad range of gram-positive, gram-negative, aerobic, anaerobic, and atypical species of bacteria, including antimicrobial-resistant strains.[6-9]

The ribosome is a common target for antimicrobials. As a result of the antimicrobial binding to the ribosomal target, protein synthesis can be inhibited with bacteriostatic or bactericidal effects. The mode of action for tetracyclines is to bind to the bacterial ribosome. But mutational changes in bacteria have given rise to resistance to tetracyclines, mainly by two mechanisms: efflux mechanisms, which pump the antibiotic out of the cell, and ribosomal protection, which interferes with binding to the receptor site. Both mechanisms may be present at the same time.[4,6,10]

Tigecycline has been shown to reversibly bind to the ribosome with a strong affinity, which may explain how it overcomes tetracycline resistance. To date, naturally occurring tigecycline-resistant strains have not been observed,[3] and attempts to create tigecycline-resistant isolates in the laboratory have not been successful.[11]

Pharmacokinetics/Pharmacodynamics

Tigecycline exhibits linear, dose-proportional pharmacokinetics.[4,8] A large volume of distribution at steady state (approximately 700 L) indicates that tigecycline is widely distributed in body tissues.[5,8,12] Nearly 22% of tigecycline is excreted in urine as unchanged drug, indicating that renal elimination is a secondary pathway of elimination.[8] In animal models, biliary excretion is high, and it is also a likely means of systemic clearance in humans.

The mean half-life of tigecycline is 36 hours,[4] and multiple-dose administration produces steady-state serum levels within a few days.[5] Gender and age do not appear to influence the pharmacokinetics of tigecycline.[13] These studies also show a postantibiotic effect of 5 hours for *Escherichia coli* strains and of 9 hours for *Streptococcus pneumoniae*.[14] Observations from in vitro studies also found long postantibiotic effects for tigecycline against isolates of *Staphylococcus aureus* (>3 hours) and *E coli* (1.8 to 2.9 hours).[15]

Table 9-1: In Vitro Activities of Tigecycline and Comparators

Organism and antimicrobial agent	MIC (µg/mL) Range	90%
Staphylococcus aureus (methicillin susceptible)		
Tigecycline	0.06-0.5	0.25
Minocycline	0.03-8	0.25
Oxacillin	0.06-2	1
Ceftriaxone	1-8	4
Vancomycin	0.5-2	1
Quinupristin/dalfopristin	0.12-1	0.5
Linezolid	1-4	4
Gatifloxacin	0.03-8	0.06
Staphylococcus aureus (methicillin resistant)		
Tigecycline	0.12-1	0.25
Minocycline	0.06-16	8
Oxacillin	4->16	>16
Ceftriaxone	4->32	>32
Vancomycin	0.5-2	1
Quinupristin/dalfopristin	0.25-1	1
Linezolid	1-4	4
Gatifloxacin	0.06-8	4

Organism and antimicrobial agent	MIC (µg/mL) Range	90%
Enterococcus faecalis		
Tigecycline	<0.015-1	0.25
Minocycline	0.03->32	16
Oxacillin	8->16	>16
Ceftriaxone	8->32	>32
Vancomycin	0.5->128	2
Quinupristin/dalfopristin	0.25->32	32
Linezolid	1-4	2
Gatifloxacin	0.12->16	16
Enterococcus faecium		
Tigecycline	0.03-0.25	0.12
Minocycline	0.06-32	16
Oxacillin	4->16	>16
Ceftriaxone	4->32	>32
Vancomycin	0.25->128	>128
Quinupristin/dalfopristin	0.25-32	4
Linezolid	1-4	2
Gatifloxacin	0.12->16	>16

(continued on next page)

Table 9-1: In Vitro Activities of Tigecycline and Comparators
(continued)

Organism and antimicrobial agent	MIC (μg/mL) Range	90%
Streptococcus pneumoniae (penicillin susceptible)		
Tigecycline	≤0.015-1	0.25
Minocycline	0.03-16	0.5
Oxacillin	≤0.03-2	0.25
Ceftriaxone	≤0.015-0.25	0.03
Vancomycin	0.12-0.5	0.5
Quinupristin/dalfopristin	0.25-1	1
Linezolid	0.25-1	1
Gatifloxacin	0.06-0.5	0.5
Streptococcus pneumoniae (penicillin resistant)		
Tigecycline	0.03-1	0.5
Minocycline	0.06-16	16
Oxacillin	0.5->16	>16
Ceftriaxone	0.25-2	1
Vancomycin	0.25-0.5	0.5
Quinupristin/dalfopristin	0.25-1	1
Linezolid	0.25-1	1
Gatifloxacin	0.12-1	0.5

Organism and antimicrobial agent	MIC (μg/mL) Range	90%
Escherichia coli		
Tigecycline	0.06-1	0.5
Minocycline	0.25-64	8
Piperacillin	0.5->128	>128
Piperacillin/tazobactam	0.25->128	4
Ceftriaxone	≤0.06-4	≤ 0.06
Imipenem	≤0.06-2	0.25
Gatifloxacin	≤0.008-16	0.5
Tobramycin	0.25-8	2
Enterobacter cloacae		
Tigecycline	0.25-4	2
Minocycline	2-32	8
Piperacillin	0.5->128	>128
Piperacillin/tazobactam	1->128	128
Ceftriaxone	≤0.06->128	>128
Imipenem	0.12-2	1
Gatifloxacin	0.015-16	0.25
Tobramycin	0.25-32	1

(continued on next page)

Table 9-1: In Vitro Activities of Tigecycline and Comparators
(continued)

Organism and antimicrobial agent	MIC (μg/mL) Range	90%
Enterobacter aerogenes		
Tigecycline	0.25-8	2
Minocycline	1-64	16
Piperacillin	2->128	>128
Piperacillin/tazobactam	1->128	128
Ceftriaxone	≤ 0.06>128	64
Imipenem	0.25-2	2
Gatifloxacin	0.03->16	>16
Tobramycin	0.25-32	16
Pseudomonas aeruginosa		
Tigecycline	0.5-32	32
Minocycline	2->64	32
Piperacillin	2->128	>128
Piperacillin/tazobactam	0.25->128	>128
Ceftriaxone	8->128	>128
Imipenem	0.25->128	32
Gatifloxacin	0.25->16	>16
Tobramycin	0.25->32	>32

(Modified from Milatovic[9])

Organism and antimicrobial agent	MIC (µg/mL) Range	90%
Acinetobacter		
Tigecycline	0.06-4	2
Minocycline	≤0.03-16	8
Piperacillin	1->128	>128
Piperacillin/tazobactam	0.06->128	>128
Ceftriaxone	0.12->128	>128
Imipenem	≤0.06->128	32
Gatifloxacin	0.03-16	16
Tobramycin	0.12->32	32
Haemophilus influenzae		
Tigecycline	0.12-2	1
Minocycline	0.12-2	1
Piperacillin	≤0.06-64	0.25
Piperacillin/tazobactam	≤0.06-0.5	≤0.06
Ceftriaxone	≤0.06-0.12	≤0.06
Imipenem	≤ 0.06-2	1
Gatifloxacin	≤ 0.008-0.06	0.015
Tobramycin	0.5-8	4

Safety and Tolerability

Three safety and tolerability studies evaluated the effects of single and multiple ascending IV doses of tigecycline in healthy subjects.[8] No serious adverse events were reported. Dose-related nausea and vomiting were the most common and are typical adverse events for the tetracycline class. Nausea was experienced by 48.5% of tigecycline recipients and vomiting by 29.4%. Both nausea and vomiting tended to increase in frequency with increasing dose.

Another study evaluated the safety of two doses of tigecycline, 25 mg and 50 mg, administered by IV every 12 hours for 7 to 14 days.[5] Nausea and vomiting were the most common adverse events, followed by diarrhea, indicating that most adverse events were gastrointestinal.

Additional Studies

An in vitro study of tigecycline activity against 1,924 clinical isolates showed that it possessed excellent activity against all gram-positive cocci tested, as well as potent effect against most Enterobacteriaceae, *Acinetobacter*, and *Stenotrophomonas*[9] (Table 9-1). Studies by Gales et al and Pachón-Ibáñez et al also indicate tigecycline has good activity against *Acinetobacter baumannii*.[16,17] Neither tigecycline nor minocycline (Dynacin®, Minocin®), however, had any clinical efficacy against *Pseudomonas aeruginosa*.

A particularly significant characteristic of tigecycline is its activity against resistant gram-positive organisms such as penicillin-resistant *S pneumoniae*, methicillin-resistant *S aureus* (MRSA), and vancomycin-resistant enterococci (VRE). These initial studies hold promise that tigecycline has low potential for the development of resistance and may be an important therapeutic option.

Telavancin

The emergence of resistant strains of enterococci and staphylococci stimulated the development of glycopeptides with improved activity and mechanisms of action.

One of these new glycopeptides under development is telavancin (TD-6424).

Telavancin (Arbelic™) is a novel, semisynthetic derivative of vancomycin (Vancocin®). It produces rapid and concentration-dependent bactericidal activity against a range of susceptible and resistant gram-positive organisms.[18-22] Studies have shown that telavancin has a broad spectrum of activity against important gram-positive organisms that cause serious infections, including methicillin-susceptible *S aureus* (MSSA) and MRSA, vancomycin-intermediate enterococci and VRE, and penicillin-susceptible and penicillin-resistant *Streptococcus pneumoniae*.[18,21,22]

Pharmacokinetic/Pharmacodynamic Properties

The pharmacokinetic/pharmacodynamic properties of an antimicrobial agent are important factors in the selection of dosing frequency for optimal effect.[23,24] Studies have identified at least two distinct mechanisms of action for telavancin that enhance early bactericidal activity and decrease the potential for resistance. One of the mechanisms is inhibition of peptidoglycan synthesis.[19-21] Compared to vancomycin, telavancin was shown to be more than 10 times as active at inhibiting peptidoglycan synthesis in MRSA and *E coli*.[20]

Telavancin was also observed to disrupt cell membrane integrity, which results in increased membrane permeability, leakage of cytoplasmic ATP and K+ ions, and depolarization of membrane potential.[19,20] A direct correlation was seen between membrane potential and bacterial viability, which suggests that this mechanism of action may be responsible for the rapid bactericidal activity of telavancin.

Studies by Hegde et al in an animal model showed that telavancin had comparable efficacy at four different dosing intervals. This is consistent with the finding that the area under the concentration-time curve/minimum inhibitory concentration (AUC/MIC) ratio was the variable that best predicted efficacy.[18]

Table 9-2: Postantibiotic Effect for Telavancin and Comparator Antibiotics

Antibiotic	PAE (hours)		
	MSSA	MRSA	GISA
Telavancin	4	6	4
Vancomycin	1	1	1
Nafcillin	0	ND	ND

MSSA, methicillin-susceptible *S aureus*; MRSA, methicillin-resistant *S aureus*; GISA, glycopeptide-intermediate *S aureus*; ND, not determined.

(Modified from Pace[21])

Pace et al found a long duration of postantibiotic effect (PAE) for telavancin (7 hours) against *S aureus* isolates, compared to a substantially shorter PAE for vancomycin and no PAE for nafcillin (Nafcil®, Unipen®, Nallpen®)[21] (Table 9-2). Additional studies demonstrated that the pharmacokinetic profile of telavancin is linear and predictable, making once-daily dosing the preferable regimen.[18,19]

Telavancin also has a high protein-binding capacity, which prolongs the elimination half-life of the agent.[25] Following the administration of doses of 1 to 15 mg/kg, the half-life for telavancin ranged from 5 to 9 hours.[19]

Safety and Tolerability

Adverse events were mild in severity when telavancin was administered by IV in doses up to 15 mg/kg/d over 30 minutes for 7 days.[19] Transient, mild taste disturbance and headache were the most commonly reported adverse events. Taste disturbance was reported by 75% of the subjects, and

40% reported headaches. Other adverse events included dizziness (35%), site reaction (25%), and nausea (20%).

In contrast to the mild adverse events experienced with telavancin, adverse events experienced with vancomycin include anaphylactoid reactions, such as urticaria, pruritus, wheezing, headache, and flushing of the head and trunk (red man syndrome).[19]

Although early clinical data found increases in the QTc interval in subjects receiving telavancin,[19] later studies by Barriere et al show telavancin had a minimal effect on QT prolongation. Investigators concluded there was a low risk of cardiac toxicity.[26]

Additional Studies

King et al compared the in vitro activity of telavancin with that of vancomycin, teicoplanin, linezolid (Zyvox®), quinupristin/dalfopristin (Synercid®), moxifloxacin (Avelox®), and an appropriate penicillin (ampicillin, penicillin, or oxacillin).[22] Telavancin was active against all gram-positive organisms tested. Results showed that telavancin appeared to be superior to other glycopeptides tested and comparable to or better than the other agents tested (Table 9-3).

A clinical study compared telavancin vs standard therapy for the treatment of complicated skin and soft-tissue infections from gram-positive bacteria.[27] The standard regimens were either antistaphylococcal penicillin four times a day or vancomycin twice a day. For patients with *S aureus* infection, 80% who were treated with telavancin were cured vs 77% of those receiving standard therapy. For patients with MRSA infection, cure rates were 82% for telavancin-treated patients and 69% for those treated with standard therapy. In addition, the MIC at which 90% of the isolates were inhibited was lower for telavancin in all *S aureus* tested and was comparable to vancomycin and oxacillin.

Goldstein et al compared telavancin in vitro with other antimicrobials against anaerobic gram-positive bacteria

Table 9-3: Comparative In Vitro Activity of Telavancin Against Selected Aerobic Gram-Positive Bacteria

Organism	Antimicrobial	MIC range	MIC90
MSSA	telavancin	0.25-1	0.5
	vancomycin	1-2	2
	teicoplanin	0.5-2	2
	linezolid	2-2	2
	quin/dalfo	0.5-1	1
	erythromycin	0.25->64	64
	moxifloxacin	0.03-0.125	0.125
	oxacillin	0.25-1	1
MRSA	telavancin	0.125-1	0.5
	vancomycin	1-2	1
	teicoplanin	0.5-16	2
	linezolid	0.5-2	2
	quin/dalfo	0.5-1	0.5
	erythromycin	0.25->64	>64
	moxifloxacin	0.03-8	4
	oxacillin	16->64	>64
E faecalis vancomycin-susceptible	telavancin	0.06-1	1
	vancomycin	0.5-2	2
	teicoplanin	0.03-0.5	0.25
	linezolid	2-4	4
	quin/dalfo	2-8	8
	erythromycin	0.125->64	>64
	ampicillin	0.5-2	2

Organism	Antimicrobial	MIC range	MIC90
E faecalis	telavancin	0.25-4	4
vancomycin-resistant	vancomycin	4->256	>256
	teicoplanin	0.06-32	32
	linezolid	1-4	4
	quin/dalfo	2-32	8
	erythromycin	0.25->64	>64
	ampicillin	1-2	2
E faecium	telavancin	0.06-0.5	0.5
vancomycin-susceptible	vancomycin	0.5-2	1
	teicoplanin	0.5-2	1
	linezolid	2-4	4
	quin/dalfo	0.25-4	2
	erythromycin	2->64	>64
	ampicillin	8-64	64
E faecium	telavancin	0.5-8	4
vancomycin-resistant	vancomycin	64->256	>256
	teicoplanin	4-64	32
	linezolid	1-2	2
	quin/dalfo	0.5-8	4
	erythromycin	2->64	>64
	ampicillin	32->256	64

(continued on next page)

Table 9-3: Comparative In Vitro Activity of Telavancin Against Selected Aerobic Gram-Positive Bacteria

(continued)

Organism	Antimicrobial	MIC range	MIC90
Streptococcus pneumoniae	telavancin	0.008-0.03	0.016
	vancomycin	0.25-0.5	0.5
	teicoplanin	0.03-0.125	0.125
	linezolid	0.5-1	1
	quin/dalfo	0.25-1	1
	erythromycin	0.06->64	64
	moxifloxacin	0.06-0.25	0.25
	penicillin	0.008-0.5	0.25

MSSA, methicillin-susceptible *S aureus*; MRSA, methicillin-resistant *S aureus*; quin/dalfo, quinupristin/dalfopristin (Modified from King[22])

and *Corynebacterium*.[28] The study demonstrated that telavancin has potent activity at <1μg/mL against a broad range of gram-positive anaerobes as well as unusual aerobes, including *Actinomyces* and *Propionibacterium* spp, *Peptostreptococcus*, *Clostridium perfringens*, *Clostridium difficile*, and *Corynebacterium*.

Dalbavancin

Similar to telavancin, dalbavancin (BI 397) is a novel semisynthetic glycopeptide for IV administration. Also similar to telavancin, dalbavancin has advantages compared to other glycopeptides, such as less-frequent dosing, more rapid bactericidal action, and less likelihood for the development of resistance.[29,30] Dalbavancin disrupts bacterial cell-wall synthesis[31] and is active against a broad range of clinically important gram-positive organisms, including staphylococci, streptococci, enterococci, corynebacteria, and anaerobes.[32-36] Dalbavancin, however, is not active against most gram-negative bacteria.[36]

Pharmacokinetics/Pharmacodynamics

A unique feature of dalbavancin is its extremely slow elimination from the body (7-12 days).[31,32,37,38] Dalbavancin is highly bound (>98%) to plasma protein, primarily albumin, which accounts for its long half-life.[32,39] Neither vancomycin nor linezolid is highly protein bound, each having a binding rate of approximately 30%.[39] Plasma concentrations of 20 mg/L are bactericidal, and studies show that doses of 500 mg or more of dalbavancin will maintain concentrations above the MIC for at least 1 week.[38] The goal of dosing regimens is to deliver safe and effective drug concentrations to the site of infection and maintain concentrations at an adequate level for an adequate period.[40]

Clinical studies by Leighton et al demonstrated dalbavancin's linear, dose-proportional pharmacokinetics[38] (Figure 9-1). These studies and those by Dorr et al[40] found that approximately one third of the dose of dalbavancin was excreted unchanged in the urine. This suggests that nonrenal routes of elimination play a role in the elimination of dalbavancin, whereas elimination for vancomycin and teicoplanin is almost exclusively via the kidneys.

Safety and Tolerability

Leighton et al assessed the tolerability, pharmacokinetics, and serum bactericidal activity of IV dalbavancin in healthy volunteers. Investigators found no serious adverse events or deaths among dalbavancin recipients. The most common adverse events were fever (50%), headache (25%), and nausea (6%). Fever was defined as any oral temperature of >37.1°C. There were no clinically significant laboratory findings or ECG changes associated with this antibiotic.

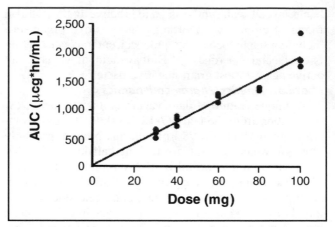

Figure 9-1: Linear regression analysis of dalbavancin following administration of single 30-min IV doses of 140 to 1,120 mg.

Additional Studies

Animal studies demonstrated that dalbavancin has good penetration into the site of infection for skin and soft-tissue infections.[39] In comparing dalbavancin to linezolid, single doses of 25 and 50 mg/kg of linezolid were expected to be effective against MSSA and MRSA, respectively, based on the pharmacokinetics of linezolid. However, doses at those levels were not effective, and a single 100 mg/kg oral dose of linezolid was necessary to achieve the same reduction in bacteria as was seen with a single 10 mg/kg IV dose of dalbavancin. In addition, when treated with linezolid, regardless of the dose, regrowth of bacteria began by 24 to 48 hours in animal models. Dalbavancin's excellent penetration and high plasma concentrations over an extended period made it a more effective therapy in this animal model.

Three dosing regimens were evaluated in a clinical study by Seltzer et al.[32] Of the 62 patients who partici-

Table 9-4: Comparator Antimicrobials Used for Treatment of Skin and Soft-Tissue Infections

Antimicrobial	No. of patients receiving drug
Ceftriaxone alone or in combination	6
Cefazolin alone or in combination	4
Piperacillin and tazobactam in combination	3
Clindamycin alone	2
Vancomycin alone or in combination	4
Linezolid alone	1
Cephalexin alone	1

Note: Comparators were determined by investigators before randomization.

(Modified from Seltzer[32])

pated in the study, 20 received a single 1,100 mg dose of dalbavancin, 21 received 1,000 mg on day 1 and 500 mg on day 8, and 21 patients received a comparator chosen by the investigators before randomization (Table 9-4). Clinical success rates at both end-of-therapy and at follow-up evaluation were more favorable for the two-dose dalbavancin group vs the single-dose and standard-of-care groups (Table 9-5). Both dalbavancin regimens were well tolerated, and most adverse events (90%) were considered to be of mild to moderate severity.

An exception to dalbavancin's potent activity against susceptible and resistant gram-positive bacteria is VRE of the Van A phenotype.[33,41] Dalbavancin was also not as effective against several *Lactobacilli*.[35]

A worldwide assessment of dalbavancin activity against more than 6,000 isolates[41] confirmed prior investigations

Table 9-5: Populations and Outcomes by Treatment Group, of Three Regimens of Treatment for Skin and Soft-Tissue Infections

Variable

Response to treatment

  Clinical success

     At end-of-therapy visit

        Intent-to-treat population

        Clinically evaluable population

     At follow-up visit

        Intent-to-treat population

        Clinically evaluable population

  Microbiologic success[a]

[a] For microbiologic success, n/N is the number of pathogens eradicated/number of pathogens detected.

(Modified from Seltzer[32])

regarding its in vitro activity.[33,36] With the exception of the Van A phenotype of VRE, all three studies found that dalbavancin demonstrated potent activity against *S aureus* (both susceptible and resistant strains), coagulase-negative *S aureus* (CoNS), and all streptococci tested, including *S pneumoniae*, β-hemolytic, and viridans group Streptococci. Dalbavancin demonstrated significantly better activity against staphylococci than did vancomycin, teicoplanin, or oritavancin.[33,36] Two different animal studies of staphylococcal endocarditis models indicated that dalbavancin is as effective as vancomycin and teicoplanin in reducing bacteria.[33,42]

Treatment group, n/N (%)		
1-dose dalbavancin	**2-dose dalbavancin**	**Comparator**
15/20 (75)	19/21 (91)	17/21 (81)
13/16 (81)	16/17 (94)	17/21 (81)
12/20 (60)	19/21 (91)	16/21 (76)
8/13 (62)	16/17 (94)	16/21 (76)
7/12 (58)	12/13 (92)	12/17 (71)

Raad et al evaluated treatment of catheter-related bloodstream infections in 75 adult patients with dalbavancin compared to vancomycin.[43] Dalbavancin treatment was a single 1,000 mg dose followed by a 500 mg dose 1 week later, and the vancomycin was administered IV twice daily for 14 days. The gram-positive bacteria isolated in the study included CoNS and *S aureus*, including MRSA. Patients treated with dalbavancin had an 87% overall success rate (range 73.2% to 100%), which was significantly higher than rates for those treated with vancomycin (50% with a 31.5% to 68.5% range).

Another study examined the ability of dalbavancin and vancomycin to prevent *S aureus* colonization of catheter devices.[44] Biofilm commonly forms around catheters, and vancomycin displays poor activity against organisms embedded within biofilm. The study showed that rates of colonization were comparable in the vancomycin- and control- (normal saline) treated groups (53% and 47%, respectively), but only 28% colonization was seen in those treated with dalbavancin. Although the lower rate of colonization following dalbavancin treatment was not statistically significant, the trend toward lower colonization indicates that dalbavancin may play a role in the prevention and treatment of device-related infection.

In addition to being well tolerated, cumulative data from studies indicate that dalbavancin's favorable pharmacokinetics support once-weekly dosing (1,000 mg on day 1 and 500 mg on day 8) and may result in better patient compliance,[40] early discharge, and possible facilitation of home IV therapy.[45]

Similar to telavancin, dalbavancin appears to be an effective option for treatment of serious skin and soft-tissue infections caused by gram-positive organisms. Dalbavancin has received priority review from the FDA and, may be available in late 2005.

Doripenem

Doripenem (S-4661) is a novel broad-spectrum parenteral carbapenem with enhanced activity against nonfermentative gram-negative bacilli.[46,47] It is also active against members of the Enterobacteriaceae family, anaerobes, and gram-positive cocci.[48]

Doripenem was discovered in Japan and is being co-developed in the United States for the treatment of hospitalized patients with serious systemic bacterial infections.[49,50] Limited animal-study and clinical-trial data have been published on doripenem, but six phase III clinical trials are in progress for complicated urinary tract infections (including pyelonephritis), complicated intra-abdominal infections, and nosocomial pneumonia (including ventilator-associated pneumonia). Phase I trials of a nebulized formulation of doripenem are also in progress for treatment of cystic fibrosis.[51]

The carbapenem class of antibiotics exhibits a wide spectrum of bactericidal activity against gram-positive and gram-negative bacteria. Carbapenem resistance, particularly in *P aeruginosa* and *Acinetobacter* strains, has emerged as a concern in some hospitals.

The emergence of resistance to carbapenems is mediated by various mechanisms, including carbapenemases, efflux pumps, and reduced cell membrane permeability through loss of OprD porins.[46,49] Because multiple mechanisms are needed for resistance to doripenem, the likelihood is low that combinations of resistance mechanisms will be selected in vivo,[52] reducing the potential for emerging resistance.

Pharmacokinetics/Pharmacodynamics

Doripenem combines features of imipenem and meropenem for a spectrum that is similar to older antipseudomonal carbapenems but has greater activity against some nonfermentative bacilli.[53] Pharmacokinetic and pharmacodynamic properties of doripenem are similar to those of meropenem.

Doripenem is β-lactamase stable, including to extended-spectrum β-lactamases (ESBLs), and is bactericidal against most species.[46,48] Doripenem has low serum protein binding (8.9%), a half-life of approximately 1 hour, and postantibiotic effects lasting nearly 2 hours in vitro for gram-negative isolates. Maximum serum concentrations of doripenem were shown to reach approximately 50 µg/mL following a 1,000 dose infused for more than 1 hour, and approximately 60% to 75% of doripenem administered IV was recovered in the urine within 24 hours.[54]

Safety and Tolerability

Similar to meropenem, doripenem is safe and well tolerated in humans, with a minimal risk of seizures.[46,54] Serious renal toxicity and neurotoxicity have been associated with carbapenems, but animal and human studies have not demonstrated this toxicity in doripenem.[48,54] The addition of cilastin to imipenem is necessary to prevent an enzyme, dehydropeptidase I (DHP-I), from breaking down imipenem and creating toxic metabolites. Doripenem is not hydrolyzed by DHP-I and does not require the addition of cilastatin.[55] However, the addition of cilastatin to doripenem improves the concentration of the antimicrobial in plasma.[48]

Additional Studies

In vitro studies found that, overall, doripenem demonstrated activity similar to that of imipenem against gram-positive isolates and similar to that of meropenem against gram-negative isolates.[50] Enterobacteriaceae with ESBLs and/or inducible or derepressed AmpC β-lactamases are not associated with increased MICs of doripenem. The MICs at which 90% of Enterobacteriaceae strains were inhibited ranged from 0.03-0.5 µg/mL, with the exception of *Proteus mirabilis*, for which the MIC90 was 1 µg/mL. Studies by Nomura[56] and Tsuji[48] reached similar conclusions (Table 9-6).

Another study demonstrated that doripenem was consistently active against Enterobacteriaceae and *Acinetobacter*, except for carbapenemase-producing strains.[51] Doripenem exhibited limited activity against enterococci, as did the other carbapenems. Carbapenemase-producing *E coli* isolates, however, showed only minor reductions in susceptibility to carbapenems.

Carbapenems are often used to treat intra-abdominal and gynecologic infections because of their activity against anaerobes.[55] Mikamo et al evaluated the in vitro activities of doripenem against major gynecologic pathogens, including *Streptococcus agalactiae*, *E coli*, *Peptostreptococcus magnus*, *Bacteroides fragilis*, and *Prevotella bivia*.[55] Doripenem was effective against all strains at MIC90 ranges from 0.0625-1 µg/mL.

Mushtaq et al assessed the activity of doripenem against *P aeruginosa* in an in vitro study.[49] Doripenem and meropenem demonstrated reduced activity against isolates with increased intrinsic resistance, but imipenem did not. The loss of OprD porin also increased the MIC for doripenem. Both of these findings indicate that doripenem is affected by efflux and OprD mechanisms of resistance. Doripenem did appear to have slightly lower MICs compared to those of meropenem for strains with increased intrinsic resistance and less propensity to select for resistant mutants than meropenem.

Two separate in vitro studies confirmed results from earlier trials that doripenem is a broad-spectrum β-lactam with activity similar to meropenem and imipenem but superior to ertapenem.[46,53] Doripenem was found to have potent activity against many clinically important gram-positive cocci and nonfermentative gram-negative bacilli, including activity against *S aureus* and *P aeruginosa*. In addition to demonstrating excellent activity against Enterobacteriaceae with ESBLs or AmpC resistance mechanisms, doripenem MICs of ≤4 µg/mL inhibited penicillin-resistant Streptococci and *Haemophilus influenzae*.

Similar to dalbavancin, doripenem is undergoing FDA review and will likely be available for clinical use later in 2005.

Future Options for Development

As resistance emerges to each new antimicrobial introduced, pharmaceutical companies are refocusing their discovery efforts on developing novel agents with new mechanisms of action. Nucleosides are one class of compounds under investigation as antibacterials.[57] Some derivatives have shown moderate to good activity against specific bacterial strains.

Table 9-6: In Vitro Activities of Doripenem and Reference Antibiotics Against Clinical Isolates

| Organism | Drug | MIC (μg/mL) | |
		Range	90%
Staphylococcus aureus			
Methicillin-susceptible	Doripenem	0.032-0.125	0.063
	Imipenem	0.016-0.032	0.032
	Meropenem	0.063-0.125	0.125
	Ceftazidime	8-16	16
Methicillin-resistant	Doripenem	4-32	16
	Imipenem	1-64	32
	Meropenem	8-32	32
	Ceftazidime	32->128	>128
Streptococcus pneumoniae			
Penicillin-susceptible	Doripenem	0.004-0.016	0.008
	Imipenem	0.004-0.008	0.008
	Meropenem	0.008-0.016	0.016
	Ceftazidime	0.125-16	2
	Penicillin	0.016-0.063	0.063
Penicillin-resistant	Doripenem	0.016-2	0.5
	Imipenem	0.008-2	0.25
	Meropenem	0.016-2	0.5
	Ceftazidime	0.125-32	32
	Penicillin	0.125-4	2

Organism	Drug	MIC (µg/mL) Range	90%
Enterococcus faecalis	Doripenem	0.5-16	4
	Imipenem	0.25-8	1
	Meropenem	1-64	8
	Ceftazidime	>128	>128
Enterococcus faecium	Doripenem	0.5->128	>128
	Imipenem	0.5->128	>128
	Meropenem	1->128	>128
	Ceftazidime	32>128	>128
Escherichia coli	Doripenem	0.016-0.032	0.032
	Imipenem	0.063-0.25	0.125
	Meropenem	0.016-0.032	0.016
	Ceftazidime	0.063-1	0.25
Klebsiella pneumoniae	Doripenem	0.032-0.125	0.063
	Imipenem	0.063-0.25	0.125
	Meropenem	0.032	0.032
	Ceftazidime	0.063-0.5	0.25
Enterobacter cloacae	Doripenem	0.032-0.125	0.063
	Imipenem	0.125-1	0.5
	Meropenem	0.016-0.125	0.063
	Ceftazidime	0.063->128	128

(continued on next page)

Table 9-6: In Vitro Activities of Doripenem and Reference Antibiotics Against Clinical Isolates
(continued)

Organism	Drug	MIC (μg/mL) Range	90%
Haemophilus influenzae	Doripenem	0.032-1	0.5
	Imipenem	0.25-16	4
	Meropenem	0.032-0.5	0.25
	Ceftazidime	0.063-0.25	0.25
Pseudomonas aeruginosa			
Imipenem-susceptible	Doripenem	0.063-8	2
	Imipenem	0.25-8	8
	Meropenem	0.032-8	2
	Ceftazidime	0.5-128	32
Imipenem-resistant	Doripenem	2-16	8
	Imipenem	16-32	32
	Meropenem	2-32	16
	Ceftazidime	1-64	64

(Modified from Tsuji[48])

Genetic engineering of bacteriophages/viruses that infect bacteria may lead to a new approach to antibacterial therapy that could circumvent drug resistance.[58] Investigators at the University of California Los Angeles discovered that bacteriophages contain genes that allow them to rapidly change their proteins to bind to different cell receptors, so phages quickly evolve new variants. The goal would be to generate proteins in the laboratory that will bind to selected molecules to create new antibiotics for treating bacterial diseases.

References

1.   Infectious Diseases Society of America report: Bad bugs, no drugs. July 2004. Page 3. Available at: http://www.fda.gov/ohrms/dockets/04s0233/04s-0233-c000005-03-IDSA-vol1.pdf. Accessed June 10, 2005.

2.   Petersen PJ, Jacobus NV, Weiss WJ, et al: In vitro and in vivo antibacterial activities of a novel glycylcycline, the 9-t-butylglycylamido derivative of minocycline (GAR-936). *Antimicrob Agents Chemother* 1999;43:738-744.

3.   Chopra I: New developments in tetracycline antibiotics: glycylcyclines and tetracycline efflux pump inhibitors. *Drug Resist Updat* 2002;5:119-125.

4.   Garrison MW, Neumiller JJ, Setter SM: Tigecycline: an investigational glycylcycline antimicrobial with activity against resistant gram-positive organisms. *Clin Ther* 2005;27:12-22.

5.   Postier RG, Green SL, Klein SR, et al: Results of a multicenter, randomized, open-label efficacy and safety study of two doses of tigecycline for complicated skin and skin-structure infections in hospitalized patients. *Clin Ther* 2004;26:704-714.

6.   Fritsche TR, Kirby JT, Jones RN: In vitro activity of tigecycline (GAR-936) tested against 11,859 recent clinical isolates associated with community-acquired respiratory tract and gram-positive cutaneous infections. *Diagn Microbiol Infect Dis* 2004;49:201-209.

7.   Nathwani D: Tigecycline: clinical evidence and formulary positioning. *Int J Antimicrob Agents* 2005;25:185-192.

8.   Muralidharan G, Micalizzi M, Speth J, et al: Pharmacokinetics of tigecycline after single and multiple doses in healthy subjects. *Antimicrob Agents Chemother* 2005;49:220-229.

9.   Milatovic D, Schmitz FJ, Verhoef J, et al: Activities of the glycylcycline tigecycline (GAR-936) against 1,924 recent European clinical bacterial isolates. *Antimicrob Agents Chemother* 2003;47:400-404.

10.   Hoellman DB, Pankuch GA, Jacobs MR, et al: Antipneumococcal activities of GAR-936 (a new glycylcycline) compared to those of nine other agents against penicillin-susceptible and -resistant pneumococci. *Antimicrob Agents Chemother* 2000;44:1085-1088.

11.   Projan SJ: Preclinical pharmacology of GAR-936, a novel glycylcycline antibacterial agent. *Pharmacotherapy* 2000;20(9 pt 2):219S-228S.

12.   Murphy TM, Deitz JM, Petersen PJ, et al: Therapeutic efficacy of GAR-936, a novel glycylcycline, in a rat model of experimental endocarditis. *Antimicrob Agents Chemother* 2000;44:3022-3027.

13.   Zhanel GG, Homenuik K, Nichol K, et al: The glycyclines: a comparative review with tetracyclines. *Drugs* 2004;64:63-88.

14.   Bradford PA: A first in class glycylcycline. *Clin Microbiol News* 2004;26:163-168.

15.   Petersen PJ, Weiss WJ, Labthavikul P: The postantibiotic effect and time-kill kinetics of the glycylcyclines, GAR-936 (TBG-MINO) and (PAM-MINO). Abstract F-132 presented at: 38th Interscience Conference Antimicrobial Agents Chemotherapy. September 24-27, 1998, San Diego, California.

16.   Gales AC, Jones RN: Antimicrobial activity and spectrum of the new glycylcycline, GAR-936 tested against 1,203 recent clinical bacterial isolates. *Diagn Microbiol Infect Dis* 2000;36:19-36.

17.   Pachón-Ibáñez ME, Jiménez-Mejías ME, Pichardo C, et al: Activity of tigecycline (GAR-936) against *Acinetobacter baumannii* strains, including those resistant to imipenem. *Antimicrob Agents Chemother* 2004;48:4479-4481.

18.   Hegde SS, Reyes N, Wiens T, et al: Pharmacodynamics of telavancin (TD-6424), a novel bactericidal agent, against gram-positive bacteria. *Antimicrob Agents Chemother* 2004;48:3043-3050.

19.   Shaw JP, Seroogy J, Kaniga K, et al: Pharmacokinetics, serum inhibitory and bactericidal activity, and safety of telavancin in healthy subjects. *Antimicrob Agents Chemother* 2005;49:195-201.

20.   Higgins DL, Chang R, Debabov DV, et al: Telavancin, a multifunctional lipoglycopeptide, disrupts both cell wall synthesis and cell membrane integrity in methicillin-resistant *Staphylococcus aureus*. *Antimicrob Agents Chemother* 2005;49:1127-1134.

21.   Pace JL, Krause K, Johnston D, et al: In vitro activity of TD-6424 against *Staphylococcus aureus*. *Antimicrob Agents Chemother* 2003;47:3602-3604.

22.   King A, Phillips I, Kaniga K: Comparative in vitro activity of telavancin (TD-6424), a rapidly bactericidal, concentration-dependent anti-infective with multiple mechanisms of action against gram-positive bacteria. *J Antimicrob Chemother* 2004;53:797-803.

23.   Craig WA: Pharmacokinetic/pharmacodynamic parameters: rationale for antibacterial dosing of mice and men. *Clin Infect Dis* 1998;26:1-10.

24.   Liu P, Muller M, Derendorf H: Rational dosing of antibiotics: the use of plasma concentrations versus tissue concentrations. *Int J Antimicrob Agents* 2002;19:285-290.

25.   Van Bambeke F: Glycopeptides in clinical development: pharmacological profile and clinical perspectives. *Curr Opin Pharmacol* 2004;4:471-478.

26.   Barriere S, Genter F, Spencer E, et al: Effects of a new antibacterial, telavancin, on cardiac repolarization (QTc interval duration) in healthy subjects. *J Clin Pharmacol* 2004;44:689-695.

27.   Stryjewski ME, O'Riordan WD, Lau WK, et al: Telavancin versus standard therapy for treatment of complicated skin and soft-tissue infections due to gram-positive bacteria. *Clin Infect Dis* 2005;40:1601-1607.

28.   Goldstein EJ, Citron DM, Merriam CV, et al: In vitro activities of the new semisynthetic glycopeptide telavancin (TD-6424), vancomycin, daptomycin, linezolid, and four comparator agents against anaerobic gram-positive species and *Corynebacterium* spp. *Antimicrob Agents Chemother* 2004;48:2149-2152.

29.   Malabarba A, Goldstein BP: Origin, structure, and activity in vitro and in vivo of dalbavancin. *J Antimicrob Chemother* 2005;55(suppl 2):ii15-ii20.

30.   Raghavan M, Linden PK: Newer treatment options for skin and soft tissue infections. *Drugs* 2004;64:1621-1642.

31.   Anderegg TR, Biedenbach DJ, Jones RN: Initial quality control evaluations for susceptibility testing of dalbavancin (BI 397), an investigational glycopeptide with potent gram-positive activity. *J Clin Microbiol* 2003;41:2795-2796.

32.   Seltzer E, Dorr MB, Goldstein BP, et al: Once-weekly dalbavancin versus standard-of-care antimicrobial regimens for treat-

ment of skin and soft-tissue infections. *Clin Infect Dis* 2003;37:1298-1303.

33.   Candiani G, Abbondi M, Borgonovi M, et al: In-vitro and in-vivo antibacterial activity of BI 397, a new semi-synthetic glycopeptide antibiotic. *J Antimicrob Chemother* 1999;44:179-192.

34.   Lopez S, Hackbarth C, Romanò G, et al: In vitro antistaphylococcal activity of dalbavancin, a novel glycopeptide. *J Antimicrob Chemother* 2005;55(suppl S2):ii21-ii24.

35.   Goldstein EJ, Citron DM, Merriam CV, et al: In vitro activities of dalbavancin and nine comparator agents against anaerobic gram-positive species and corynebacteria. *Antimicrob Agents Chemother* 2003;47:1968-1971.

36.   Jones RN, Biedenbach DJ, Johnson DM, et al: In vitro evaluation of BI 397, a novel glycopeptide antimicrobial agent. *J Chemother* 2001;13:244-254.

37.   Guay DR: Dalbavancin: an investigational glycopeptide. *Expert Rev Anti Infect Ther* 2004;2:845-852.

38.   Leighton A, Gottlieb AB, Dorr MB, et al: Tolerability, pharmacokinetics, and serum bactericidal activity of intravenous dalbavancin in healthy volunteers. *Antimicrob Agents Chemother* 2004;48:940-945.

39.   Jabés D, Candiani G, Romanó G, et al: Efficacy of dalbavancin against methicillin-resistant *Staphylococcus aureus* in the rat granuloma pouch infection model. *Antimicrob Agents Chemother* 2004;48:1118-1123.

40.   Dorr MB, Jabes D, Cavaleri M, et al: Human pharmacokinetics and rationale for once-weekly dosing of dalbavancin, a semi-synthetic glycopeptide. *J Antimicrob Chemother* 2005;55(suppl S2):ii25-ii1130.

41.   Streit JM, Fritsche TR, Sader HS, et al: Worldwide assessment of dalbavancin activity and spectrum against over 6,000 clinical isolates. *Diagn Microbiol Infect Dis* 2004;48:137-143.

42.   Lefort A, Pavie J, Garry L, et al: Activities of dalbavancin in vitro and in a rabbit model of experimental endocarditis due to *Staphylococcus aureus* with or without reduced susceptibility to vancomycin and teicoplanin. *Antimicrob Agents Chemother* 2004;48:1061-1064.

43.   Raad I, Darouiche R, Vazquez J, et al: Efficacy and safety of weekly dalbavancin therapy for catheter-related bloodstream in-

fection caused by gram-positive pathogens. *Clin Infect Dis* 2005;40:374-380.

44. Darouiche RO, Mansouri MD: Dalbavancin compared with vancomycin for prevention of *Staphylococcus aureus* colonization of devices in vivo. *J Infect* 2005;50:206-209.

45. Mushtaq S, Warner M, Johnson AP, et al: Activity of dalbavancin against staphylococci and streptococci, assessed by BSAC and NCCLS agar dilution methods. *J Antimicrob Chemother* 2004;54:617-620.

46. Jones RN, Huynh HK, Biedenbach DJ: Activities of doripenem (S-4661) against drug-resistant clinical pathogens. *Antimicrob Agents Chemother* 2004;48:3136-3140.

47. Iso Y, Irie T, Nishino K, et al: A novel 1 beta-methylcarbapenem antibiotic, S-4661. Synthesis and structure-activity relationships of 2-(5-substituted pyrrolidin-3-ylthio)-1 beta-methylcarbapenems. *J Antibiot* (Tokyo) 1996;49:199-209.

48. Tsuji M, Ishii Y, Ohno A, et al: In vitro and in vivo antibacterial activities of S-4661, a new carbapenem. *Antimicrob Agents Chemother* 1998;42:94-99.

49. Mushtaq S, Ge Y, Livermore DM: Doripenem versus *Pseudomonas aeruginosa* in vitro. activity against characterized isolates, mutants, and transconjugants and resistance selection potential. *Antimicrob Agents Chemother* 2004;48:3086-3092.

50. Ge Y, Wikler MA, Sahm DF, et al: In vitro antimicrobial activity of doripenem, a new carbapenem. *Antimicrob Agents Chemother* 2004;48:1384-1396.

51. Mushtaq S, Ge Y, Livermore DM: Comparative activities of doripenem versus isolates, mutants, and transconjugants of Enterobacteriaceae and *Acinetobacter* spp. with characterized β-lactamases. *Antimicrob Agents Chemother* 2004;48:1313-1319.

52. Livermore DM: Of *Pseudomonas*, porins, pumps and carbapenems. *J Antimicrob Chemother* 2001;47:247-250.

53. Jones RN, Huynh HK, Biedenbach DJ, et al: Doripenem (S-4661), a novel carbapenem: comparative activity against contemporary pathogens including bactericidal action and preliminary in vitro methods evaluations. *J Antimicrob Chemother* 2004;54:144-154.

54. Thye DA, Kilfoil T, Leighton A, et al: Abstract A-21 presented at: 43rd Interscience Conference Antimicrobial Agents Chemotherapy. September 14-17, 2003, Chicago, Illinois.

55. Mikamo H, Izumi K, Hua YX, et al: In vitro and in vivo antibacterial activities of a new injectable carbapenem, S-4661, against gynaecological pathogens. *J Antimicrob Chemother* 2000;46:471-474.

56. Nomura S, Nagayama A: In vitro antibacterial activity of S-4661, a new parenteral carbapenem, against urological pathogens isolated from patients with complicated urinary tract infections. *J Chemother* 2002;14:155-160.

57. Rachakonda S, Cartee L: Challenges in antimicrobial drug discovery and the potential of nucleoside antibiotics. *Curr Med Chem* 2004;11:775-793.

58. U.S. Department of Health and Human Services. National Institutes of Health. Scientists discover potential new way to control drug-resistant bacteria. NIH News. September 23, 2004. Available at: http://www.nih.gov/news/pr/sep2004/niaid-22.htm. Accessed June 14, 2005.

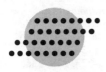

Index

H

Haemophilus influenzae 23-25, 27, 56, 58, 60, 180, 188, 235, 251, 254
  type B 56
headache 83, 110, 112, 238, 243
heart disease 158
Helicobacter 7
hemodialysis 31, 100, 101
hemolysin 96
Herellea vaginicola 123
Hiprex® 16
HIV 55, 107, 181
HMG-CoA reductase inhibitors 107
hypotension 72, 83, 158

I

imipenem 15, 21, 32, 33, 94, 122, 129, 137, 138, 140-142, 150, 154, 162, 164, 167-169, 177, 181, 182, 185, 193, 219, 233-235, 249-254
imipenem/cilastatin (Primaxin®) 15, 138, 139, 141, 165, 166, 191-193
impetigo 81, 82, 83
indinavir 107
interferon 72
Invanz® 15, 168
isoniazid (Nydrazid®) 11

J

joint infections 31, 57, 106, 148, 157, 185, 190, 196

K

kanamycin (Kantrex®) 11
Kantrex® 11

Kawasaki syndrome 71
Keflex® 14
Keflin® 14
Kefzol® 14, 87, 219
keratitis 190, 196
Ketek™ 13
ketolides 26
Klebsiella 180, 219
Klebsiella pneumoniae 7, 21, 25, 26, 58, 102, 137, 219, 253

L

Lactobacilli 245
leukocytosis 158
leukopenia 158
Levaquin® 25, 61, 142, 168, 194
levofloxacin (Levaquin®) 23-27, 32, 33, 61, 76, 142, 150, 162, 164, 168, 169, 185, 191, 194
lidocaine 107
Lincocin® 13
lincomycin (Lincocin®) 13
lincosamides 13
linezolid (Zyvox®) 16, 17, 60, 84, 85, 87, 104, 105, 108-111, 230-232, 239-241, 243-245
lipopeptides 85, 112
Listeria 6
Lorabid® 14
loracarbef (Lorabid®) 14
lovastatin 107

M

Macrobid® 16, 105, 168
Macrodantin® 16, 105
macrolides 12, 26, 28, 29, 63, 76, 94

271